Respiratory Disease Series: Diagnostic Tools and Disease Managements

Series Editors

Hiroyuki Nakamura
Ibaraki Medical Center
Tokyo Medical University
Ibaraki
Japan

Kazutetsu Aoshiba
Ibaraki Medical Center
Tokyo Medical University
Ibaraki
Japan

This book series cover a variety of topics in respiratory diseases, with each volume providing an overview of the current state of knowledge, recent discoveries and future prospects for each disease. In each chapter the editors pose critical questions, which are often unresolved clinical issues. These are then discussed by the authors, providing insights and suggestions as to which developments need to be addressed. The series offers new information, which will inspire innovative ideas to further develop respiratory medicine.This collection of monographs is aimed at benefiting patients across the globe suffering from respiratory disease.
Edited by established authorities in the field and written by pioneering experts, this book series will be valuable to those researchers and physicians working in respiratory medicine. The series is aimed at a broad readership, and the books will also be a valuable resource for radiologists, emergency medicine physicians, pathologists, pharmacologists and basic research scientists.

More information about this series at http://www.springer.com/series/15152

Keisaku Fujimoto
Editor

Disaster and Respiratory Diseases

Springer

Editor
Keisaku Fujimoto
Clinical Laboratory Sciences
Shinshu University School of Health Science
Matsumoto
Nagano
Japan

ISSN 2509-5552 ISSN 2509-5560 (electronic)
Respiratory Disease Series: Diagnostic Tools and Disease Managements
ISBN 978-981-13-2597-7 ISBN 978-981-13-2598-4 (eBook)
https://doi.org/10.1007/978-981-13-2598-4

Library of Congress Control Number: 2018961565

This Springer imprint is published by Springer Nature, under the registered company Springer Nature Singapore Pte Ltd.
The registered company address is: 152 Beach Road, #21-01/04 Gateway East, Singapore 189721, Singapore

Preface

Disasters, such as earthquakes, tsunamis, volcanic eruptions, floods, typhoons, tornadoes, sediment disasters and accidents, not only cause injury and death but also induce respiratory diseases, such as respiratory infections, and aggravate chronic lung diseases, such as chronic obstructive pulmonary disease (COPD) and asthma, following the deterioration of the environment. This e-book is part of a series describing respiratory diseases and issues related to disasters as well as measurements during or after a disaster based on experiences in Japan.

As Japan is located at the intersection of a marine plate and continental plate, it is susceptible to earthquakes, and large-scale damage can occur due to tsunamis following such earthquakes because the country is surrounded by the sea and has long shorelines. Furthermore, Japan is located in the Circum-Pacific belt, with 108 active volcanoes equivalent to approximately 7% of the total on the planet. Therefore, natural disasters, such as earthquakes, tsunamis and volcanic eruptions, can occur frequently, with the Great Hanshin Awaji Earthquake Disaster, East Japan Great Earthquake Disaster, the Kumamoto Earthquake and the eruptions of Mt. Ontakesan and Shiranesan as recent examples. It has been reported that approximately one third of patients conveyed to a disaster centre hospital at the time of the East Japan Great Earthquake Disaster were diagnosed with respiratory diseases. The tsunami caused by the earthquake disaster, the poor residential environment and poor hygiene just after the earthquake disaster, air pollution and the shortage of medical supplies led to the onset of pneumonia and aggravation of COPD and asthma. Furthermore, the daily living in a car after the earthquake disaster caused a number of deaths due to pulmonary thromboembolism caused by deep vein thrombosis. Patients prescribed long-term oxygen therapy (LTOT), called home oxygen therapy (HOT) in Japan, did not have access to oxygen supply equipment because of damage and power outages, and large numbers of such patients rushed to medical institutions for oxygen supply resulting in panic.

Therefore, the outbreak, aggravation and exacerbation of respiratory diseases are important problems at the time of the disaster. However, there have been few reports regarding the problems, measurement and prevention of the onset and aggravation of respiratory diseases at the time of and following a large-scale disaster. Therefore, it is important to share the experience and know-how gained in Japan with the world.

Health-related problems at the time of a large-scale disaster outbreak are as follows: (1) lung injury induced directly by the disaster; (2) onset of respiratory infection, pulmonary thromboembolism due to deep vein thrombosis and aggravation of existing lung diseases related to deterioration of residential environment and environmental hygiene; (3) aggravation of existing respiratory diseases by the lack of health resources due to power outages or lifeline stoppage; (4) lifeline stoppage, and the measurements and preparation for a disaster by patients publicly and patients themselves are important.

Matsumoto, Japan Keisaku Fujimoto

Contents

Part I
Respiratory Injury Directly Induced by a Disaster

Chapter 1
Dust, Asbestos, and Sludge Exposure: What Kinds of Respiratory Injuries Are Caused by Disaster-Induced Dust, Asbestos, and Sludge Exposure?

Shinya Ohkouchi, Shinsuke Yamanda, Shu Hisata, Masao Tabata, Toshiya Irokawa, Hiromasa Ogawa, and Hajime Kurosawa

Abstract In past disasters, marked increases in the frequencies of common respiratory diseases, such as community-acquired pneumonia, and the exacerbation of chronic obstructive pulmonary disease and bronchial asthma were observed. The temporary deterioration of the health status of the general public due to problems with infrastructure and health management systems was probably responsible for these increases. On the other hand, no significant increases in the incidence rates of conditions caused by damage to the peripheral respiratory system or asbestosis have been reported in large populations that experienced disasters.

The reason for this is unclear; however, the following hypothesis is reasonable: (1) The chemical and physiological characteristics, size, and density of inhaled particles have a significant influence on the incidence rates of respiratory conditions. (2) Most inhaled dust becomes caught in the upper respiratory tract; therefore, damage to the peripheral respiratory tract is uncommon.

Thus, pulmonary injuries tend to affect the health of rescue team members, construction workers, and volunteers, who handle large amounts of dust and/or sludge. Pulmonary injuries often result in serious and/or fatal outcomes. Therefore, suitable protective regulations are required, even under the confusing situations found after disasters. Accordingly, it will be necessary to establish standard methods for the use

S. Ohkouchi (✉) · M. Tabata · T. Irokawa · H. Ogawa · H. Kurosawa
Occupational Health and Respiratory Medicine, Graduate School of Medicine, Tohoku University, Sendai, Japan
e-mail: ohkouchi@rm.med.tohoku.ac.jp

S. Yamanda
Department of Respiratory Medicine, Sendai Kousei Hospital, Sendai, Japan

S. Hisata
Respiratory Medicine, Jichi Medical University, Shimotsuke, Japan

K. Fujimoto (ed.), *Disaster and Respiratory Diseases*,
Respiratory Disease Series: Diagnostic Tools and Disease Managements,
https://doi.org/10.1007/978-981-13-2598-4_1

of respiratory protective equipment and the evaluation of the risk of respiratory conditions in disaster zones. In addition, it might be possible to predict the risk of malignant mesothelioma (including due to asbestosis) after disasters that cause buildings to collapse. Careful longitudinal observation is needed for the early diagnosis of mesothelioma.

In this section, we introduce the conditions in which peripheral pulmonary damage can occur and some case reports involving pulmonary injuries. In addition, we discuss ways in which lung damage can be avoided in future disasters.

Keywords Respiratory injuries · Asbestosis · Disaster · Protection · Great East Japan Earthquake

1.1 Introduction

1.1.1 Natural Disasters and Respiratory Conditions

Disasters can be classified into man-made and natural disasters. Man-made disasters include fires, explosions, building collapses, chemical accidents, etc. and can be caused by conscious or unconscious actions. Natural disasters include earthquakes, volcano eruptions, storms, floods, tsunamis, etc. [1, 2].

The respiratory system is very sensitive to the effects of disasters because it is affected by the inhalation and aspiration of harmful particles, vapors, liquids, near-drowning, respiratory burns, etc. [3–5]. Respiratory injuries can be caused by various incidents, such as those described above, and such injuries are not clearly defined. The term "respiratory injuries" includes various entities, such as acute and chronic conditions; central and peripheral conditions; infectious and noninfectious conditions; and pleural, arterial, vascular, lymphatic, airway conditions, etc. [6, 7].

All survivors of disasters are at increased risk of respiratory conditions. These conditions reflect the post-disaster situation, for example, overcrowding can lead to respiratory infections [8].

In this section, we mention that respiratory injuries, mainly diffuse lung disease (DLD), can be caused by exposure to large amounts of dust, asbestos, or sludge after natural disasters (based on the findings of previous studies and our experience of the Great East Japan Earthquake).

1.1.2 Respiratory Injuries and Diffuse Lung Disease (DLD)

To understand the respiratory injuries caused by disaster-related particle inhalation, it is important to consider the physiological and chemical characteristics, sizes, and quantities of the particles. Generally, respiratory infections and the exacerbation of chronic obstructive pulmonary disease (COPD) and bronchial asthma (BA) occur much more frequently than DLD after natural disasters [9–12]. On the other hand, DLD can be fatal. Therefore, it is very important to protect healthy workers from these diseases to avoid unnecessary deaths. After natural disasters, DLD tends to be seen in rescue team members and construction workers because they work in grimy environments [12–15]. Generally, the effects of asbestos derived from buildings that are destroyed in disasters are not obvious [16–18]. In this section, we mainly focus on our experiences of DLD and asbestosis in Japan and propose preventative measures that could reduce the risk of lung injuries after disasters. Acute respiratory distress syndrome (ARDS) differs from DLD because the definition of ARDS is based on localized edema and the PaO_2/FiO_2 (partial pressure of oxygen in arterial blood/fraction of inspired oxygen); however, a wide range of lung injuries are observed in ARDS patients.

1.1.3 The Great East Japan Earthquake

The Great East Japan Earthquake in 2011 (magnitude: 9.0) was the strongest in history, and the epicenter was located in the Japan Trench in the Pacific Ocean. This earthquake caused a tsunami, which killed a significant number of people within several minutes of the earthquake. The National Police Agency of Japan reported that the disaster killed 15,894 people and that 2562 people remained missing as of February 10, 2016. Of these deaths, 91%, 4%, and 1% were due to drowning, injuries caused by debris or other elements, and fire, respectively. In addition, hypothermia from exposure to cold seawater and/or weather might have contributed to the fatalities. Furthermore, 55.7% of those who died were over 65 years old. Rescue teams were unable to approach the affected coastal regions for several days because of repeated tsunamis, and most patients that required intensive care were unable to reach emergency rooms [19].

The Great East Japan Earthquake damaged lots of infrastructure (e.g., the electricity grid, including nuclear power plants; water, oil, and natural gas supplies; and communication and transport systems), which was not repaired for weeks or months and caused a deterioration of public hygiene in the disaster zone. In addition, approximately 0.5 million people were evacuated into overcrowded shelters after the disaster, which coincided with a period of cold weather [8, 20]. The occurrence rates of respiratory infections, such as community-acquired pneumonia and influenza, and the exacerbation of BA or COPD were two to three times higher than normal in all age groups in the disaster zone [8–10]. On the other hand, no significant increases in the frequencies of acute or chronic DLD were observed [8–10]. A few reports about DLD in residents of the disaster zone or workers involved in the removal of dust/sludge from the disaster zone will be introduced in the case reports section. No increase in the frequency of asbestosis had been observed in this population by the end of 2017.

1.2 Disaster Categories and DLD

1.2.1 Fire-Related Respiratory Injuries

Many disasters, such as earthquakes, wildfires, and thunderstorms, cause fires. Fire-related deaths only accounted for 1% of all deaths in the Great East Japan Earthquake. However, in the Great Hanshin Earthquake in 1995, fire accounted for almost 10% of deaths [21]. The two earthquakes caused different types of damage, which is considered to be explained by the earthquakes' characteristics. The Great East Japan Earthquake (magnitude: 9.0) predominantly involved the horizontal oscillation of a slipping continental plate for a long period (3 min), and the epicenter was located in the Japan Trench, which is about 100 km from mainland Japan in the Pacific Ocean. Therefore, a huge tsunami developed and damaged coastal areas, but it caused relatively little damage to buildings and relatively few fires in comparison with the Great Hanshin Earthquake. The Great Hanshin Earthquake (magnitude: 7.3) predominantly involved the pitching and strong oscillation of the ground right below Kobe for a short period (15 s). There was no tsunami, but many buildings collapsed in a limited area [22]. Acute smoke inhalation and thermal bronchial injuries can cause asphyxia and ARDS. In the case of the St Helens volcano eruption, two cases of ARDS due to thermal and inhalation injuries were reported [23].

The mortality rate of burn cases increases from 4% to around 30% if inhalation injuries are present [24]. Direct thermal injuries to the upper airway are common, but such injuries rarely affect the lower airway [25]. Smoke contains various respiratory irritants (carbonaceous particulates, sulfur oxides, nitrogen oxides, phenols, formaldehyde, vapor acids, alkalis, etc.), which cause mucosal inflammation, including of the peripheral alveolar epithelial cells, and ARDS [26]. Poorly water-soluble substances can also cause delayed injuries up to 48 h after exposure. In addition, the absorption of systemic toxins, such as carbon monoxide and hydrogen cyanide, which are generated through incomplete combustion, can result in the impairment of oxygen delivery and cellular respiration [27].

The manifestations of acute smoke inhalation injuries can take several hours to appear. Repeated chest X-ray or chest computed tomography (CT) examinations are required to detect pulmonary edema/ARDS. Bronchoscopy is useful for the early detection and evaluation of the degree of mucosal damage. Early intubation should be considered to avoid airway obstruction and to allow appropriate airway management to be initiated at an early stage. The nebulization of adrenaline and corticosteroids has been used to try and minimize airway edema although there is no conclusive evidence of the efficacy of this approach [1, 25].

1.2.2 Building Collapses

Various disasters, including earthquakes, tsunamis, tornados, landslides, accidents, and terrorist attacks, can cause buildings to collapse, which leads to dust, sludge, and asbestos being released from the building. In dry and windy climates, the dust is spread and reduces air quality in wide areas. The effects of inhaled particles on the respiratory system were investigated in detail in the case of the attack on the World Trade Center (the WTC attack) [3, 5, 12, 28–30].

Immediately after the WTC attack, the dust released by the collapse of the buildings and the combustion of jet fuel produced a dense and intensely toxic atmospheric plume. The highly alkaline dust produced in this incident induced bronchial hyperreactivity and/or a persistent cough (WTC cough) and exacerbated asthma [5]. On the other hand, no significant increases in the frequencies of DLD or asbestosis-related disease have been detected since the disaster (at the end of 2017), even among populations who directly inhaled the toxic plume [3, 12, 28]. The populations at greatest risk of exposure included firefighters, the police, paramedics, other first responders, construction workers, and volunteers, who participated in the initial rescue and recovery operation and then spent many months clearing rubble. Antao et al. suggested that protective respiratory masks, including type 1 (full-face respirators), type 2 (half-face respirators), type 3 (disposable masks with N95 to P100 ratings), and type 4 (other disposable masks) masks, reduced the frequency of respiratory symptoms and respiratory diseases in the short term; however, there were no differences in effectiveness among the four mask types [29]. It is still unclear whether respiratory protective equipment helps to protect against the small particles and harmful gasses that cause DLD and ARDS [28]. In some cases, such as accidents or explosions at chemical plants, the use of more strict respiratory protective equipment, such as face shields for air-feeding masks, might be necessary [4]. There are work environment-dependent regulations about mask use by construction workers in many countries, but there is no evidence that mask use helps to protect against DLD or asbestosis [31–33]. Occupational health specialists will need to establish adequate procedures for protecting against lung injuries caused by environmental factors after disasters.

Similarly, there are few case reports about acute or chronic lung injuries associated with the WTC attack [5]. This seems to be explained by (1) the use of respiratory protective equipment and (2) the fact that particles of smaller than 10 μm, which can reach the alveolar spaces, exhibited low frequencies among the dust released by the attack (<2%). The standard particle size encountered after the WTC attack was >50 μm. However, huge quantities of particles (a "soup of dust") measuring >10 μm were found in lungs of firefighters [3, 28, 34].

In the Great Hanshin Earthquake and the Great East Japan Earthquake, several cases of DLD due to the inhalation of dust or sludge, involving rescue team members or construction workers, were reported. These diseases included acute interstitial pneumonia (AIP) and organizing pneumonia (OP) [35–38]. Pulmonary alveolar proteinosis (PAP) and acute eosinophilic pneumonia (AEP) are caused by lung injuries involving the small airways, and disaster-related case reports of PAP and AEP can be found in PubMed [34, 39, 40]. Inadequate use of respiratory protective equipment was observed in these cases. Some of these cases are summarized in the case report section in this review.

1.2.3 Trauma

When buildings collapse, the associated traumas can cause ARDS. In addition, pulmonary embolisms and pneumonia can complicate chest traumas, and ARDS and renal failure can develop in patients with severe polytrauma or crush injuries [1, 41]. The majority of patients that suffer disaster-related traumas are admitted to hospital in the first 24 h [41, 42]. The very young and the very old are at highest risk of trauma-related mortality [43]. Chest trauma is seen in around 10% of earthquake casualties who present to hospital, and the management of such cases can be complicated by delays of several hours or days in rescuing wounded people from the rubble [44]. Chest injuries are often accompanied by injuries to other organ systems, and multiple injuries are associated with increased mortality. Accidents in which patients become trapped or engulfed or in which objects drop onto them can cause crush syndrome, which can induce renal failure due to blood clotting and changes in the compositions of bodily fluids. Crush syndrome can also cause ARDS and multiple organ failure. In the Great Hanshin Earthquake, 10% (around 500 people) of all deaths could have been prevented if crush syndrome had been treated with dialysis [44]. To reduce the frequency of respiratory death due to ARDS, it is necessary to prevent multiple organ failure and crush syndrome.

1.2.4 Asbestosis

The two major types of asbestos, chrysotile (white asbestos) and crocidolite (blue asbestos), were used as heat shield materials for the construction of buildings until the 1970s because large amounts of asbestos are available in the natural environment and mining it is easy. Asbestos is composed of long and thin fibers with a diameter of a few micrometers. Asbestos fibers can reach the parietal pleura from inspired air by passing through the peripheral alveoli. There are no procedures for removing asbestos from the parietal pleura. Asbestos in the parietal pleura, especially crocidolite, results in continuous scraping, oxidative stress, and inflammation in the peripheral pleura during respiration. Eventually, the asbestos can cause malignant mesothelioma [3, 16, 28, 45]. The use of asbestos in construction was prohibited or limited under very strict regulations in many countries from the 1970s onward, as it causes many health problems, deaths, and legal actions. There are many large old buildings containing asbestos around the world. The widespread destruction of these buildings due to natural disasters, war, or terrorism can contaminate the environment. In particular, rescue teams, sludge cleanup teams, and construction workers without knowledge of how asbestos should be handled can be exposed to air polluted with asbestos. The adequate use of powered air-purifying respirators, protective clothing, and wetting methods could prevent the occurrence of asbestosis, including malignant mesothelioma [31, 32].

To the best of our knowledge, there have not been any reports about significant increases in the incidence of malignant mesothelioma induced by the inhalation of asbestos after disasters. However, the future risk of mesothelioma should be considered over several decades because malignant mesothelioma exhibits a long latency period in humans [5]. There have already been some reports and press releases about malignant mesothelioma arising in workers or volunteers who participated in the recovery operations after the WTC collapse or the Great Hanshin Earthquake. The establishment and thorough enforcement of measures that prevent such individuals from inhaling asbestos will be needed in future disasters.

1.2.5 Aspiration and Near-Drowning

A sudden rise in water levels, such as during a tsunami, hurricane, or flood, can cause drowning, aspiration, and trauma. Such incidents can lead to the catastrophic disruption of infrastructure and the deterioration of sanitation levels in the medium to long term. The aspiration of water into the lungs can lead to infections, alveolar surfactant loss, pulmonary edema, and ARDS [46]. Pulmonary edema is more common after immersion in salt water than after immersion in fresh water [47]. In addition, the vomiting of swallowed water can lead to the aspiration of gastric contents, especially if consciousness and/or protective airway reflexes are impaired [47]. In the 2004 Indian Ocean Earthquake and the subsequent tsunami, near-drownings, and traumas accounted for most of the immediate post-disaster morbidity. One medical team reported the cases of 37 patients who had aspirated soil-contaminated salt water. Around half of these patients developed aspiration pneumonia, and eight patients developed ARDS. Pneumothorax (19%) and pneumomediastinum (8%) also occurred as a later complication in those receiving ventilatory support [48, 49]. Fungal infections can also complicate near-drowning and should be considered in patients who do not respond to antibacterial therapy, patients who develop pneumonia or ARDS after acute aspiration, and patients who develop brain abscesses or meningitis [50, 51]. Mold or fungus can contaminate wet buildings following hurricanes or floods, causing respiratory illness in susceptible individuals [1].

1.3 Case Reports

1.3.1 Acute Interstitial Pneumonia (AIP)

There have been a few reports about AIP after natural disasters. Ohkouchi et al. reported the case of a 61-year-old male, who was engaged in making wood chips from wooden debris from the Great East Japan Earthquake and died from AIP [36]. He usually made wood chips for biomass power generation from scrap wood from dismantled buildings (under the strict regulation of environmental laws) [52].

However, he made wood chips from contaminated wood derived from the tsunami sludge from the disaster zone for few months after the Great East Japan Earthquake. The tsunami sludge contained huge amounts of unknown impurities derived from various human activities, the soil, and the seabed. He used sealed masks; however, he occasionally removed his mask because wearing it was unpleasant. A few times, he accidentally crashed into contaminated mold-infested cob walls and cans containing unknown chemicals in farmhouses. At 2 months after the earthquake, he experienced shortness of breath and was diagnosed with bacterial pneumonia at a general physician's clinic. Antibiotics were not effective, and his hypoxemia progressed. Then, he visited a pulmonary specialist at 3 months after the earthquake and was admitted to a university hospital. His chest radiographic and CT findings revealed an elevating diaphragm during inspiration and traction bronchiectasis combined with consolidation, primarily in the bilateral lower dorsal lung field, which was suggestive of fatal lung damage. Significant restrictive impairment was observed in a pulmonary function test (his vital capacity was markedly reduced). We diagnosed him with AIP based on a surgical lung biopsy examination. Despite treatment with steroid therapy, including methylprednisolone pulse therapy, immunosuppressive drugs, anticoagulants, endotoxin hemodiafiltration, and mechanical ventilation, he died 4 months after the earthquake. An autopsy confirmed the presence of AIP. We concluded that the inhalation of harmful materials from the wooden debris might have caused an acute lung injury that subsequently led to AIP (Fig. 1.1).

1.3.2 Organizing Pneumonia (OP)

Yamanda et al. reported the cases of two patients (58-year-old and 63-year-old males) with OP who engaged in restoration work to remove tsunami sludge [37]. They visited a hospital about 2 months after the Great East Japan Earthquake and were diagnosed with OP based on surgical biopsy examinations. Pathological analyses revealed multifocal peribronchiolitis and OP. In addition, electron probe microanalysis (EPMA) of these specimens demonstrated the presence of elements from the earth's crust in the inflammatory lesions. Therefore, the authors concluded that the inhalation of particles derived from tsunami sludge can cause OP. These patients recovered after the administration of corticosteroids (Fig. 1.2). Cases of OP involving construction workers who took part in restoration work after other disasters, such as the Miyake-Jima volcano eruption, the 2004 Chuetsu Earthquake, and the collapse of the WTC, have also been reported, and these patients recovered after corticosteroid therapy [12, 34, 53–55].

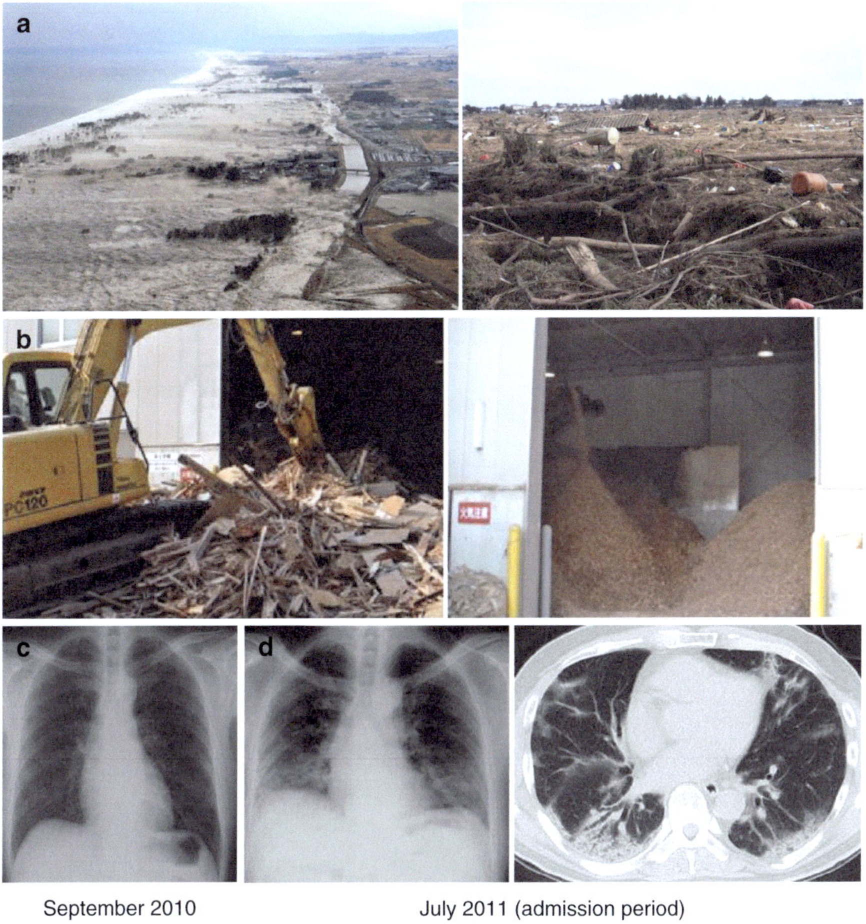

Fig. 1.1 A case of acute interstitial pneumonia in a worker making chips from wooden debris generated by the Great East Japan earthquake and tsunami. (**a**) The destructive tsunami hits East coast of the main island of Japan (left). Massive debris including unknown substances covered the damaged areas (right). (**b**) The wooden chips were generated from wooden waste using heavy equipment (left) and a shredder (right). In a typical situation, wooden waste is separated from contaminants. However, immediately after the disaster, the waste included high levels of impurities. (**c**) His chest radiographs taken before the onset of disease were mostly normal. (**d**) The chest radiograph (left) and computed tomographic scan (right) taken at admission revealed reduced lung volume, predominantly dorsal consolidation in both lungs, and traction bronchiectasis. These findings suggest serious acute lung injury. (**e**) The clinical course after admission. The various treatments applied were ineffective

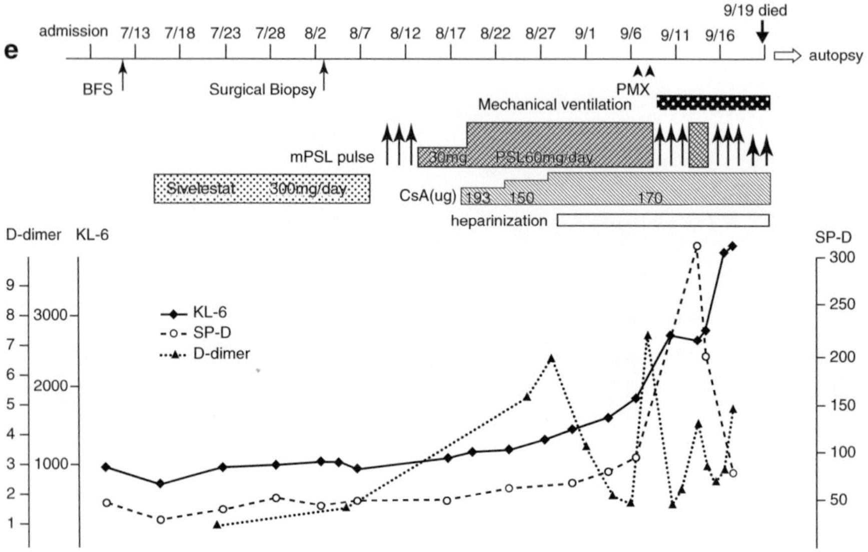

Fig. 1.1 (continued)

1.3.3 Pulmonary Alveolar Proteinosis (PAP)

Alveolar macrophages can become dysfunctional after they ingest dust-derived extraneous materials in the alveolar spaces, which can cause PAP. In many cases of PAP, autoantibodies against granulocyte-macrophage colony-stimulating factor (GM-CSF) have been detected in serum and bronchial alveolar lavage fluid (BALF). Previous studies have shown that acute and chronic dust exposures induce the production of autoantibodies against GM-CSF and PAP. In some acute onset cases or earlier cases involving steroid use, autoantibodies against GM-CSF might not be detected [56, 57].

Hisata et al. reported a case (involving a 63-year-old female) that was diagnosed as PAP [39]. The patient's house was destroyed by a tsunami, and she repeatedly visited her house, which was dusty, to clean it up without wearing a mask. Three weeks after the earthquake, she complained of a dry cough, and chest CT showed diffusely distributed lesions exhibiting ground glass opacity in the subpleural region. The initial analysis of her BALF and a transbronchial lung biopsy (TBLB) examination did not indicate PAP or provide helpful diagnostic information. EPMA analysis of the TBLB sample showed that her lung tissue included particles consisting of silicon, oxide aluminum, and other unknown materials. Under a clinical suspicion of idiopathic interstitial pneumonia, she was treated with prednisolone, cyclosporin, and methylprednisolone pulse therapy; however, her condition deteriorated. Eight months later, she was admitted to another hospital and under-

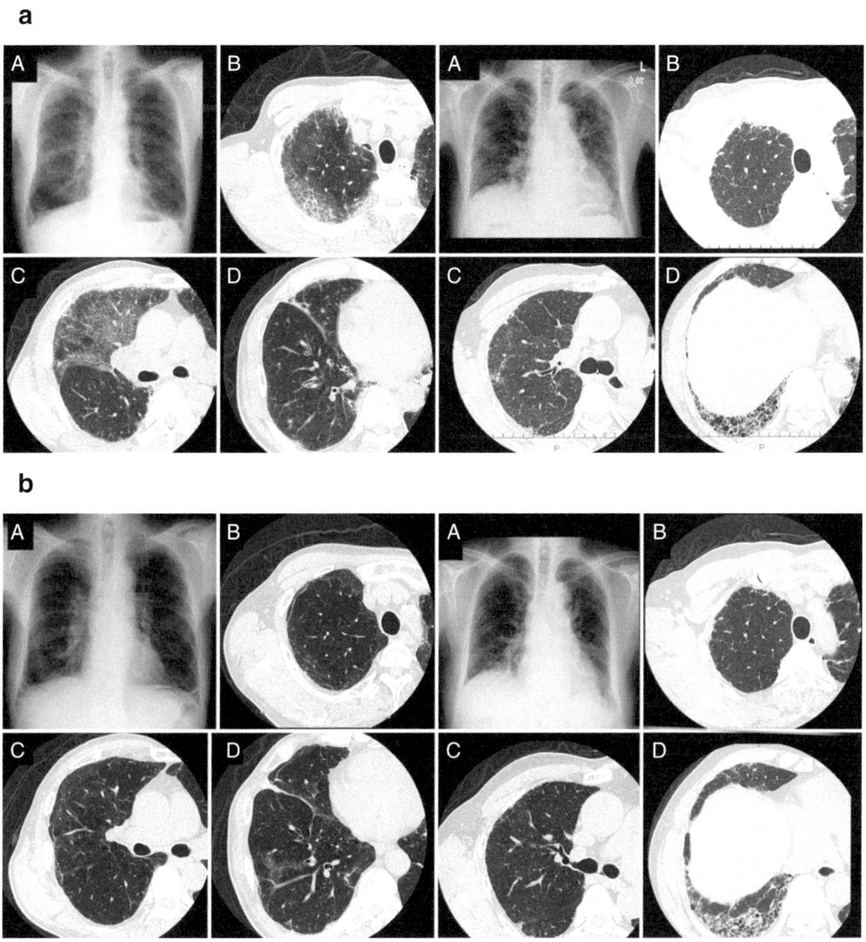

Fig. 1.2 Two cases of organizing pneumonia in a worker engaging in the restoration work after the Great East Japan earthquake and tsunami. (**a**) Chest radiograph and high-resolution chest computed tomography scan in case 1 (left) and case 2 (right) before treatment. Their diagnoses were done by the surgical lung biopsy. (**b**) Chest radiograph and high-resolution chest computed tomography scan in case 1 (left) and case 2 (right) after treatment. Oral administration of prednisolone was very effective to two patients

went bronchoscopy. Her BALF had a milky appearance, which was suggestive of PAP. The patient did not exhibit an elevated level of autoantibodies against GM-CSF, and so she was diagnosed with secondary PAP. Bilateral whole lung lavage improved her condition. The authors concluded that the inhalation of tsunami sludge had induced the onset of secondary PAP (Fig. 1.3). The possibility that corticosteroids might worsen PAP was mentioned in some reports [58].

Tanino et al. reported that the number of patients with PAP, including autoimmune PAP and secondary PAP, was increased in Fukushima Prefecture, Japan, which was one of the areas that was most damaged by the tsunami caused by the Great East Japan Earthquake [40]. They presumed that the dusty environments in the areas affected by the tsunami had caused the increase in the frequency of

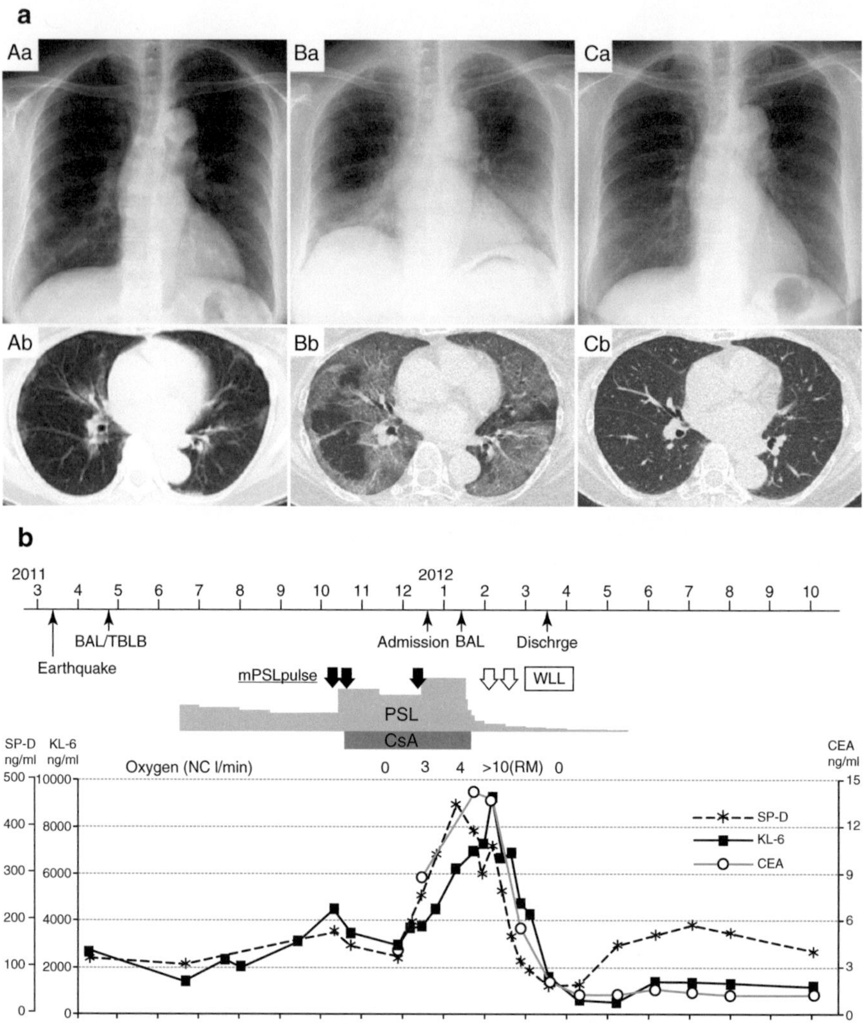

Fig. 1.3 A case of alveolar proteinosis in a resident of the destructive house by the Great East Japan earthquake and tsunami. (**A**) Chest radiograph (*a*) and computed tomography (*b*) at April 2011, January 2012, and August 2012 (left, middle, and right). (**B**) At May 2011, the diagnosis based on bronchial alveolar lavage/transbronchial lung biopsy (BAL/TBLB) was nonspecific interstitial pneumonia; however the treatment using prednisolone was not effective. At January 2012, the diagnosis was done as alveolar proteinosis based on a characteristic image and the analysis of BAL. Then, the severity of the disease was reduced dramatically by whole lung lavage (WLL)

PAP. PAP occurred in a construction worker who participated in the recovery effort after the Great Hanshin Earthquake in Kobe, 1995 [35]. The lung tissue damage seen in PAP is generally quite severe. In some reports, it has been hypothesized that exudative substances have protective effects against lung injuries in PAP.

1.3.4 Acute Eosinophilic Pneumonia (AEP)

Rom et al. reported a case of AEP in a firefighter (a 38-year-old male) exposed to high concentrations of WTC dust. He participated in the rescue work from September 11 to 24, 2001 [34]. He sometimes took off his respiratory protective equipment due to the discomfort it caused. He developed shortness of breath due to hypoxia and visited a hospital on September 24, 2001. CT showed patchy areas of ground glass density, thickened bronchial walls, and bilateral pleural effusion. His BALF demonstrated an eosinophil frequency of 70%, whereas the eosinophil frequency of his peripheral blood was only 1%, and so he was diagnosed with AEP. The administration of oxygen and corticosteroids was effective, and the patient's disease was cured without any disturbances. In his BALF, a high number of asbestos fibers had been phagocytized by macrophages, and significant quantities of fly ash and degraded fibrous glass were found. The authors concluded that the high density of dust had caused the patient's condition.

1.4 Respiratory Protective Equipment (RPE)

Proper use of respiratory protective equipment (RPE) protects the workers from the inhalation of harmful particles, vapors, and liquids in the working places [31–33]. Many kinds of RPE corresponding to various situations in working places are

Table 1.1 Reference materials of respiratory protective equipments (RPEs)

	File name	Issuing authority or company
USA	Assigned protection factors for the revised respiratory protection standard	Occupational Safety and health Administration
	https://www.3m.com/3M/en_US/safety-centers-of-expertise-us/respiratory-protection/	3M Co., Ltd.
UK	Respiratory protective equipment at work. A practical guide	Health and Safety Executive
Japan	http://www.fesc.or.jp/cfasdm/english.html	Council of Fire Appliances Standards for Disaster Management
	http://www.koken-ltd.co.jp/english/product/safe/industrial/	Koken Co., Ltd.
	http://www.sts-japan.com/global.html	Shigematsu Co., Ltd.

Table 1.2 Various respiratory protective equipments (RPEs) and the characteristics

Respiratory protective equipments (RPEs)			Assigned protection factor (APF)	Particle	Gas/vapor	
Particulate respirators	Disposable		3–10	○	×	×
	Reusable	Half face		○	×	×
		Full face	4–50	○	×	×
Powered air-purifying respirators	Half face		4–50	○	×	×
	Full face		4–100	○	×	×
	Hood type		4–25	○	×	×
	Face shield type		4–25	○	×	×
Supplied air respirators	Demand type	Half face	10	○	△	△
		Full face	50	○	△	△
	Constant flow type	Half face	50	○	△	○
		Full face	100	○	△	○
		Hood type	25	○	○	○
		Face shield type	25	○	△	○
	Pressure demand type	Half face	50	○	△	○
		Full face	1000	○	△	○
Breathing apparatus	Demand type	Half face	10	○	△	△
		Full face	50	○	△	△
	Pressure demand type full face		5000	○	△	○
Chemical cartridge respirators	With filter		Unknown	×	○	×
	Without filter		Unknown	△	○	×

(1) This table is based on Japan Industrial Standards (JIS) T8150. See the specific low or rule in each country. (2) PF = Concentration of harmful materials on environment (outside mask)/concentration of harmful materials on inhalation (inside mask). APFs are provided by regulatory authorities. (3) Chemical Cartridge Respirators need the specific cartridge according to each gas/vapor

released from the companies. In many countries, the RPE with authorization by official organization are recommended for the industrial uses (Table 1.1). Operation supervisors should evaluate working environment about physical and chemical characters, size, the concentration of particles or vapors, etc. and select adequate RPE by reference to the assigned protection factor (APF) and/or chemical cartridge before recovery works (Table 1.2 and Fig. 1.4a). APF generally represent the efficacy of reducing of the concentration of the particles. Operation supervisors should keep the environment standards for workers published from local government with adequate RPE even under emergency situations [33]. If the evaluation of environment is not enough, the use of supplied air respirators or breathing apparatus is considered (Fig. 1.4a). In Japan, wearing of powered air-purifying respirators (PAPR) is recommended in particle environments because of the higher APF and the comfort to wear in comparison with other RPE (Fig. 1.4b).

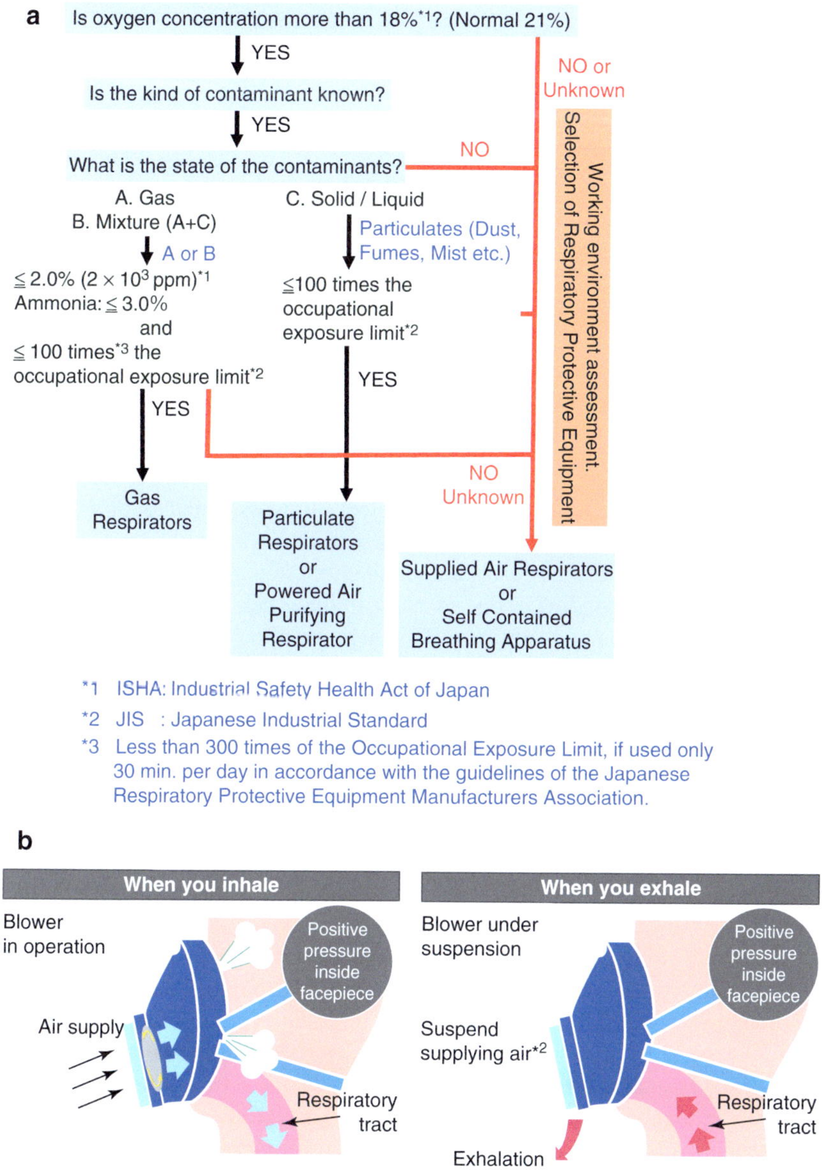

Fig. 1.4 Selection of respiratory protective equipment (RPE) in accordance with specific situation of work place. (**a**) Flowchart of RPE selection based on Japanese standards or rules. In addition, working environment assessment including atmosphere oxygen concentration, particles, gas, and characters of harmful substances before restoration work are ideal. This figure was based on the documents given from Shigematsu Works Co., Ltd., Tokyo. (**b**) The powered air-purifying respirators (PAPR) can reduce the discomfort of respiration under the masks because PPAR assist the inspiration of workers with positive pressure generated by electric fan within PPAR. Further, positive pressure prevents the contamination of particle efficiency when workers exhale. This figure was based on the documents given from Koken Co., Ltd., Tokyo

1.5 Conclusion

Pulmonary inhalation injuries are caused by the inhalation of chemical vapors, particulates, or the products of incomplete combustion [2, 4]. The clinical effects of these substances are influenced by the exposure period and the dose, solubility, and/or size of the causative agent. Highly soluble compounds and larger particles (>10 μm) primarily affect the upper airway, causing rapid symptom onset. Intermediately soluble agents and intermediate-sized particulates (5–10 μm) mainly damage the region between the larynx and segmental bronchi but can also cause parenchymal injuries, particularly when present in high concentrations. The smallest bronchi, bronchioles, and alveoli are affected by poorly soluble compounds of <5 μm in diameter [3, 28].

The respiratory system is affected by disasters because they increase the chances of the aspiration of exogenous materials and gasses, including harmful chemicals and pathogens. The following classification, which consists of phases, has been proposed to ensure that adequate measures to protect survivors of natural disasters from such diseases are taken. Phase 1, or the impact (acute) phase (lasting 0–4 days), is the period when survivors are rescued and the initial treatments for disaster-related conditions are provided. ARDS due to chest trauma, thermal injuries, crush syndrome, or the inhalation of chemical vapors might be observed in this period. Phase 2, the post-impact phase (4 days to 4 weeks), is when the first waves of infectious disease (airborne, foodborne, or waterborne infections) might emerge. ARDS due to near-drowning or aspiration pneumonia; community-acquired pneumonia; respiratory viruses, such as influenza infections (in winter); or AEP can occur in this period. Finally, phase 3, the recovery phase (after 4 weeks), is the period when DLD, including interstitial pneumonia, can develop [59, 60]. Pulmonary malignancies, including malignant mesothelioma, might not arise for several decades after a disaster [16]. The preventative effects of respiratory protective equipment against DLD and malignancy are still unknown at present [28]. The use of powered air-purifying respirators, protective clothing, and wetting methods in people who work in the affected areas are suitable for protecting against hazardous respiratory diseases; however, these measures might interfere with the swift rescuing of survivors and the rebuilding of affected areas, and they are also expensive [33]. Furthermore, vaccinations against diseases such as influenza, tuberculosis, and streptococcus pneumonia might reduce the frequency of hazardous respiratory diseases [1, 8]. Investigations into the abovementioned issues by concerned public health personnel will be needed.

References

1. Robinson B, Alatas MF, Robertson A, Steer H. Natural disasters and the lung. Respirology. 2011;16:386–95. https://doi.org/10.1111/j.1440-1843.2011.01923.x.
2. Young S, Balluz L, Malilay J. Natural and technologic hazardous material releases during and after natural disasters: a review. Sci Total Environ. 2004;322:3–20. https://doi.org/10.1016/s0048-9697(03)00446-7.

3. Lioy PJ, et al. Characterization of the dust/smoke aerosol that settled east of the World Trade Center (WTC) in lower Manhattan after the collapse of the WTC 11 September 2001. Environ Health Perspect. 2002;110:703–14.
4. Summerhill EM, et al. An official American Thoracic Society Workshop Report: chemical inhalational disasters. Biology of lung injury, development of novel therapeutics, and medical preparedness. Ann Am Thorac Soc. 2017;14:1060–72. https://doi.org/10.1513/AnnalsATS.201704-297WS.
5. Landrigan PJ, et al. Health and environmental consequences of the world trade center disaster. Environ Health Perspect. 2004;112:731–9.
6. Ranieri VM, et al. Acute respiratory distress syndrome: the Berlin Definition. JAMA. 2012;307:2526–33. https://doi.org/10.1001/jama.2012.5669.
7. Tasaka S, Tatsumi K. Clinical practice of acute respiratory distress syndrome in Japan: a nationwide survey and scientific evidences. Respir Investig. 2017;55:257–63. https://doi.org/10.1016/j.resinv.2017.04.003.
8. Ohkouchi S, et al. Deterioration in regional health status after the acute phase of a great disaster: respiratory physicians' experiences of the Great East Japan Earthquake. Respir Investig. 2013;51:50–5. https://doi.org/10.1016/j.resinv.2012.12.003.
9. Kobayashi S, et al. Impact of a large-scale natural disaster on patients with chronic obstructive pulmonary disease: the aftermath of the 2011 Great East Japan Earthquake. Respir Investig. 2013;51:17–23. https://doi.org/10.1016/j.resinv.2012.10.004.
10. Yamanda S, et al. The impact of the 2011 Great East Japan Earthquake on hospitalisation for respiratory disease in a rapidly aging society: a retrospective descriptive and cross-sectional study at the disaster base hospital in Ishinomaki. BMJ Open. 3:2013. https://doi.org/10.1136/bmjopen-2012-000865.
11. Takakura R, et al. Follow-up after the Hanshin-Awaji earthquake: diverse influences on pneumonia, bronchial asthma, peptic ulcer and diabetes mellitus. Intern Med. 1997;36:87–91.
12. Wu M, et al. Case report: lung disease in World Trade Center responders exposed to dust and smoke: carbon nanotubes found in the lungs of World Trade Center patients and dust samples. Environ Health Perspect. 2010;118:499–504. https://doi.org/10.1289/ehp.0901159.
13. Spadafora R. Firefighter safety and health issues at the World Trade Center site. Am J Ind Med. 2002;42:532–8. https://doi.org/10.1002/ajim.10153.
14. Wisnivesky JP, et al. Persistence of multiple illnesses in World Trade Center rescue and recovery workers: a cohort study. Lancet. 2011;378:888–97. https://doi.org/10.1016/s0140-6736(11)61180-x.
15. Alper HE, Yu S, Stellman SD, Brackbill RM. Injury, intense dust exposure, and chronic disease among survivors of the World Trade Center terrorist attacks of September 11, 2001. Inj Epidemiol. 2017;4:17. https://doi.org/10.1186/s40621-017-0115-x.
16. Nolan RP, et al. Risk assessment for asbestos-related cancer from the 9/11 attack on the World Trade Center. J Occup Environ Med. 2005;47:817–25.
17. Aldrich TK, et al. Lung function in rescue workers at the World Trade Center after 7 years. N Engl J Med. 2010;362:1263–72. https://doi.org/10.1056/NEJMoa0910087.
18. Friedman SM, et al. Case-control study of lung function in World Trade Center Health Registry area residents and workers. Am J Respir Crit Care Med. 2011;184:582–9. https://doi.org/10.1164/rccm.201011-1909OC.
19. Fuse A, et al. Medical relief activities conducted by Nippon Medical School in the acute phase of the Great East Japan Earthquake 2011. *J Nippon Med Sch.* 2011;78:397–400.
20. Kobayashi S, Hanagama M, Yamanda S, Yanai M. Home oxygen therapy during natural disasters: lessons from the great East Japan earthquake. Eur Respir J. 2012;39:1047–8. https://doi.org/10.1183/09031936.00149111.
21. Nakamori Y, et al. Burn injuries in the 1995 Hanshin-Awaji earthquake. Burns. 1997;23:319–22.
22. Johnson AT. Respirator masks protect health but impact performance: a review. J Biol Eng. 2016;10:4. https://doi.org/10.1186/s13036-016-0025-4.
23. Parshley PF, et al. Pyroclastic flow injury. Mount St. Helens, May 18, 1980. Am J Surg. 1982;143:565–8.

24. Smith DL, et al. Effect of inhalation injury, burn size, and age on mortality: a study of 1447 consecutive burn patients. J Trauma. 1994;37:655–9.
25. Marko P, Layon AJ, Caruso L, Mozingo DW, Gabrielli A. Burn injuries. Curr Opin Anaesthesiol. 2003;16:183–91.
26. Silva L, et al. Acute respiratory distress syndrome in burn patients: incidence and risk factor analysis. Ann Burns Fire Disasters. 2016;29:178–82.
27. Endorf FW, Gamelli RL. Inhalation injury, pulmonary perturbations, and fluid resuscitation. J Burn Care Res. 2007;28:80–3. https://doi.org/10.1097/bcr.0b013e31802c889f.
28. Lippmann M, Cohen MD, Chen L-C. Health effects of World Trade Center (WTC) dust: an unprecedented disaster with inadequate risk management. Crit Rev Toxicol. 2015;45:492–530. https://doi.org/10.3109/10408444.2015.1044601.
29. Antao VC, et al. Respiratory protective equipment, mask use, and respiratory outcomes among World Trade Center rescue and recovery workers. Am J Ind Med. 2011;54:897–905. https://doi.org/10.1002/ajim.21009.
30. Prezant DJ, et al. Cough and bronchial responsiveness in firefighters at the World Trade Center site. N Engl J Med. 2002;347:806–15. https://doi.org/10.1056/NEJMoa021300.
31. Janssen L, Zhuang Z, Shaffer R. Criteria for the collection of useful respirator performance data in the workplace. J Occup Environ Hyg. 2014;11:218–26. https://doi.org/10.1080/15459624.2013.852282.
32. Sirianni G, Borak J. How clean is "clean"? Regulations and standards for workplace clothing and personal protective equipment. J Occup Environ Med. 2010;52:190–6. https://doi.org/10.1097/JOM.0b013e3181cc55e1.
33. Goldyn SR, Condos R, Rom WN. The burden of exposure-related diffuse lung disease. Semin Respir Crit Care Med. 2008;29:591–602. https://doi.org/10.1055/s-0028-1101269.
34. Rom WN, et al. Acute eosinophilic pneumonia in a New York City firefighter exposed to World Trade Center dust. Am J Respir Crit Care Med. 2002;166:797–800. https://doi.org/10.1164/rccm.200206-576OC.
35. Tsuchiya T, Nishimura Y, Kotani Y. Secondary pulmonary alveolar proteinosis in a patient engaged in building demolition work. J Japn Respir Soc. 1999;37:219–23.
36. Ohkouchi S, et al. Fatal acute interstitial pneumonia in a worker making chips from wooden debris generated by the Great East Japan earthquake and tsunami. Respir Investig. 2012;50:129–34. https://doi.org/10.1016/j.resinv.2012.09.001.
37. Yamanda S, et al. Two cases of tsunami dust pneumonia: organizing pneumonia caused by the inhalation of dried tsunami sludge after the 2011 Great East Japan Earthquake. *Intern Med.* 2016;55:3645–53. https://doi.org/10.2169/internalmedicine.55.6952.
38. Takuma H, et al. Case report; organizing pneumonia secondary to inhalation of dried tsunami sludge after Great East Japan Earthquake. *Nihon Naika Gakkai Zasshi*. 2012;101:2307–9.
39. Hisata S, et al. Development of pulmonary alveolar proteinosis following exposure to dust after the Great East Japan Earthquake. Respir Investig. 2013;51:212–6. https://doi.org/10.1016/j.resinv.2013.04.005.
40. Tanino Y, et al. Increase in autoimmune pulmonary alveolar proteinosis after the 2011 Fukushima disaster. Allergol Int. 2016;65:332–3. https://doi.org/10.1016/j.alit.2015.12.005.
41. Gautschi OP, Cadosch D, Rajan G, Zellweger R. Earthquakes and trauma: review of triage and injury-specific, immediate care. Prehosp Disaster Med. 2008;23:195–201.
42. Bulut M, et al. Medical experience of a university hospital in Turkey after the 1999 Marmara earthquake. Emerg Med J. 2005;22:494–8. https://doi.org/10.1136/emj.2004.016295.
43. Liang NJ, et al. Disaster epidemiology and medical response in the Chi-Chi earthquake in Taiwan. Ann Emerg Med. 2001;38:549–55. https://doi.org/10.1067/mem.2001.118999.
44. Yoshimura N, et al. Profile of chest injuries arising from the 1995 southern Hyogo Prefecture earthquake. Chest. 1996;110:759–61.
45. Suzuki Y, Yuen SR. Asbestos fibers contributing to the induction of human malignant mesothelioma. Ann N Y Acad Sci. 2002;982:160–76.
46. Bierens JJ, Knape JT, Gelissen HP. Drowning. Curr Opin Crit Care. 2002;8:578–86.

47. van Berkel M, et al. Pulmonary oedema, pneumonia and mortality in submersion victims; a retrospective study in 125 patients. Intensive Care Med. 1996;22:101–7.
48. Kongsaengdao S, Bunnag S, Siriwiwattnakul N. Treatment of survivors after the tsunami. N Engl J Med. 2005;352:2654–5. https://doi.org/10.1056/nejm200506233522523.
49. Kateruttanakul P, et al. Respiratory complication of tsunami victims in Phuket and Phang-Nga. J Med Assoc Thai. 2005;88:754–8.
50. Nakamura Y, et al. Multiple Scedosporium apiospermum abscesses in a woman survivor of a tsunami in northeastern Japan: a case report. J Med Case Rep. 2011;5:526. https://doi.org/10.1186/1752-1947-5-526.
51. Nakamura Y, et al. Scedosporium aurantiacum brain abscess after near-drowning in a survivor of a tsunami in Japan. Respir Investig. 2013;51:207–11. https://doi.org/10.1016/j.resinv.2013.07.001.
52. Rohr AC, et al. Potential occupational exposures and health risks associated with biomass-based power generation. Int J Environ Res Public Health. 2015;12:8542–605. https://doi.org/10.3390/ijerph120708542.
53. Shojima J, et al. A case of volcanic ash lung: report of a case. Nihon Kokyuki Gakkai Zasshi. 2006;44:192–6.
54. Tanaka H, et al. Workplace-related chronic cough on a mushroom farm. Chest. 2002;122:1080–5.
55. Izbicki G, et al. World Trade Center "sarcoid-like" granulomatous pulmonary disease in New York City Fire Department rescue workers. Chest. 2007;131:1414–23. https://doi.org/10.1378/chest.06-2114.
56. Ohkouchi S, et al. Sequential granulocyte-macrophage colony-stimulating factor inhalation after whole-lung lavage for pulmonary alveolar proteinosis. A report of five intractable cases. Ann Am Thorac Soc. 2017;14:1298–304. https://doi.org/10.1513/AnnalsATS.201611-892BC.
57. Ono M, et al. Pathological features of explant lungs with fibrosis in autoimmune pulmonary alveolar proteinosis. Respirol Case Rep. 2017;5:e00255. https://doi.org/10.1002/rcr2.255.
58. Akasaka K, et al. Outcome of corticosteroid administration in autoimmune pulmonary alveolar proteinosis: a retrospective cohort study. BMC Pulm Med. 2015;15:88. https://doi.org/10.1186/s12890-015-0085-0.
59. Kouadio IK, Aljunid S, Kamigaki T, Hammad K, Oshitani H. Infectious diseases following natural disasters: prevention and control measures. Expert Rev Anti-Infect Ther. 2012;10:95–104. https://doi.org/10.1586/eri.11.155.
60. Aghababian RV, Teuscher J. Infectious diseases following major disasters. Ann Emerg Med. 1992;21:362–7.

Chapter 2
Tsunami Lung in Great East Japan Earthquake 2011: Clinical Time Course, Feature, Pathogenesis, and Treatment

Kohei Yamauchi, Hiromi Nagashima, Toshihide Nakadate, and Yutaka Nakamura

Abstract Drowning was the cause of death in almost all victims of the Great East Japan Earthquake Tsunami (GEJET). People who experienced near-drowning suffered from Tsunami lung afterward. Tsunami lung is initiated by the aspiration of a vast amount of sea water including sand, sludge from the sea bottom, small pieces of wood, petroleum, and undefined chemicals. Physical and chemical insults on the pulmonary tissues can cause ARDS. Subsequently, pulmonary complications by infection with microorganisms occur. The pneumonia in Tsunami lung caused by multiple pathogens including fungi was often refractory to treatment. In GEJET, *Scedosporium* species were one of the pathogens identified in patients with Tsunami lung.

Keywords Tsunami lung · Drowning · ARDS · Aspiration pneumonia · *Scedosporium* · Great East Japan Earthquake

K. Yamauchi (✉)
Division of Pulmonary Medicine, Allergy and Rheumatology, Department of Internal Medicine, Iwate Medical University School of Medicine, Morioka, Japan

Central Takizawa Hospital, Takizawa, Japan
e-mail: takakoji@herb.ocn.ne.jp

H. Nagashima · T. Nakadate
Division of Pulmonary Medicine, Allergy and Rheumatology, Department of Internal Medicine, Iwate Medical University School of Medicine, Morioka, Japan

Y. Nakamura
Department of Allergy and Rheumatology, Nippon Medical School, Graduate School of Medicine, Tokyo, Japan

K. Fujimoto (ed.), *Disaster and Respiratory Diseases*,
Respiratory Disease Series: Diagnostic Tools and Disease Managements,
https://doi.org/10.1007/978-981-13-2598-4_2

2.1 Introduction

"Tsunami lung" was firstly described after the Sumatra-Andaman tsunami in 2004 [1–3]. Medical teams from outside and clinicians in local hospitals found pulmonary complications evaluated by chest radiograph and computed tomography in the patients rescued from near-drowning conditions.

We also found patients with Tsunami lung on the Sanriku seacoast in 2011, similar condition of the patients reported as "Tsunami lung" in Sumatra disaster in 2004. Nearly 20,000 people died or went missing in the tsunami disaster following the Great East Japan Earthquake that occurred on March 11, 2011. Almost all casualties were caused by the tsunami or flooding of rivers. Victims aspirated sea water that included microorganisms from the sludge of the sea bottom, as well as sand and chemicals in the leaked heavy oil. These various materials caused severe lung damage and pulmonary infections, called "Tsunami lung" [4, 5].

2.2 Tsunami Lung in GEJET

2.2.1 Circumstances of Onset

The causes of death in the victims of the Great East Japan Earthquake Tsunami (GEJET) were mainly drowning by Tsunami waves followed by the earthquake. More than 90% of 15,870 victims were killed by the drowning (Fig. 2.1) [6]. Considering the number of victims and the patients with Tsunami lung reported, a small number of people near-drowning were fortunately rescued, but they had a risk of Tsunami lung after admission. The common background of the patients with Tsunami lung was the aspiration of more or less sea water when they were overwhelmed by Tsunami waves. As shown in Fig. 2.2, the patients of near-drowning were admitted within 24 h to Iwate Prefectural Ofunato hospital which was undamaged due to being built at the relatively higher place despite the location being very near to the area heavily damaged by tsunami. While some patients were transported to the hospital by ambulances or cars under supports of families and neighbors, a few walked by themselves to the hospital to take medical treatment. The sea water they aspirated was not usual clear sea water, but muddy black sea water containing sludge raised up from sea bottom, sand, small pieces of wood, petroleum, and undefined chemicals. Patients with Tsunami lung were basically admitted to local central hospitals such as Iwate Prefectural Ofunato hospital which were equipped with ICU. The patients with severe condition of Tsunami lung were transported by helicopters to Iwate Medical University Hospital in Morioka which is the prefectural capitol at a distance of about 100 km from Sanriku sea coast.

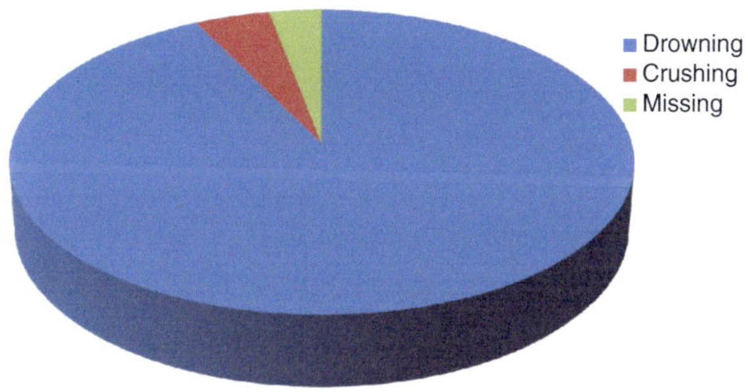

Fig. 2.1 Causes of death in the Great East Japan Earthquake 2011. Autopsy report for Iwate, Miyagi, and Fukushima Prefectures from May 11 to April 11 by Japanese National Police Agency

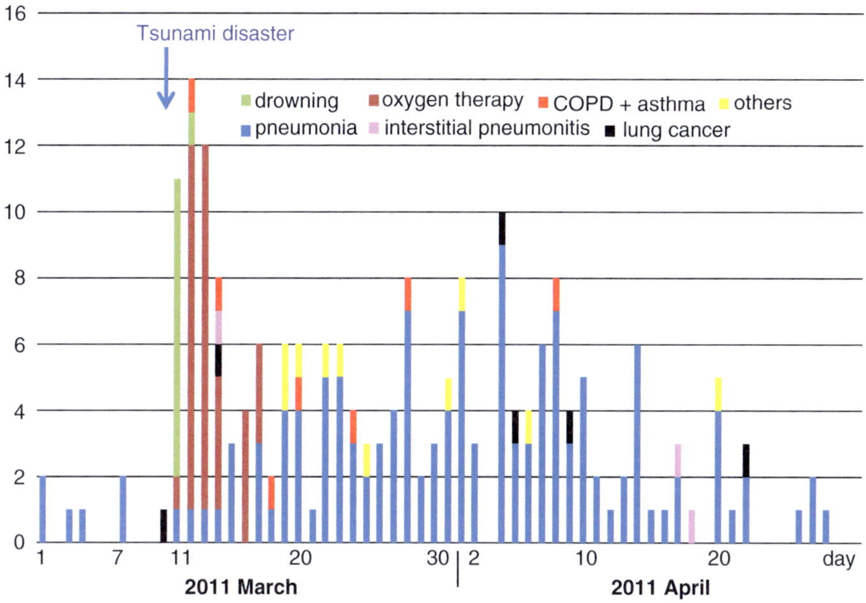

Fig. 2.2 Changes of patients with respiratory diseases admitted to Ofunato Hospital. Numbers of patients admitted to Ofunato Hospital were recorded from March 1 to April 30, 2011

2.2.2 Clinical Time Course and Features

We experienced several cases of Tsunami lung and can summarize the common feature of this disease as the following: After drowning, adult respiratory distress syndrome (ARDS) occurred by aspiration of sea water, chemicals, and various particles in an early stage of a severe case. Two or three days after drowning, pneumonia was caused by aspirated bacteria among various severities of Tsunami lung. Pneumonia of Tsunami lung was refractory to usual antibiotics in some cases. Two or three weeks later after drowning, mycotic infection might become evident as an abscess in lung and brain.

We present several severe cases of Tsunami lung who were admitted to Iwate Medical University Hospital RCU [4, 7, 8].

2.2.2.1 Case 1

A 68-year-old woman had been overwhelmed by tsunami waves was transported to a coastal clinic by the rescue team. Her chief symptom was shortness of breath after paroxysmal coughing and was transferred to a neighboring local central hospital because of low oxygen saturation (67% on 10 L/min of supplemental oxygen) as determined by pulse oximetry. A physical examination upon admission revealed a body temperature of 33.5 °C, blood pressure of 92/46 mmHg, and a regular pulse of 75 beats per minute. No evidence of trauma or fractures anywhere on her body were found. Coarse crackles were audible in both lungs. Despite confusion, a neurologic examination indicated negative findings. The laboratory findings were as follows: white blood cell count (WBC) and hemoglobin content (Hb) were within normal range; platelet counts (plt) were low as $85x10^9$ cells/L (reference range, 13.0–34.0 × 10^{10} cells/L); aspartate aminotransferase (AST), 2140 IU/L (8–40 IU/L); alanine aminotransferase (ALT), 748 IU/L(5–35 IU/L); and lactate dehydrogenase (LDH), 1160 IU/L (121–226 IU/L) were markedly high. C-reactive protein test was negative. Arterial gas analysis showed severe hypoxemia (pH 7.25; $PaCO_2$ 45 Torr; PaO_2 41 Torr) even though 10 L/min of supplemental oxygen was being administered.

A chest X-ray revealed diffuse infiltration in both lung fields. On the basis of these findings, the patient was diagnosed with aspiration pneumonia due to near-drowning.

Treatment was started with antibiotics for pulmonary infection and steroid pulse therapy for ARDS. Responding to initial treatment, she seemed to improve her general condition; however, on hospital day 26, CT scans showed pleural effusion and multiple nodular lesions in both sides (Fig. 2.3a), and the level of (1–3)-β-D-glucan (βDG) had increased to 123.4 pg/mL(0–20 pg/mL). Fungal lung disease was suspected, and treatment with 150 mg of micafungin intravenously once a day was initiated. In spite of antifungal drug, βDG increased, and brain magnetic resonance imaging (MRI) showed intraventricular abscesses (Fig. 2.3b). Since refractory mycotic infection to micafungin was suggested, micafungin was switched to voriconazole. Then after, serum βDG level gradually decreased, and pulmonary and CNS lesions were improved.

2.2.2.2 Case 2

A healthy 59-year-old woman was overwhelmed by the tsunami in the Sanriku coast. She aspirated sea water contaminated with soil and heavy oil. She swam back

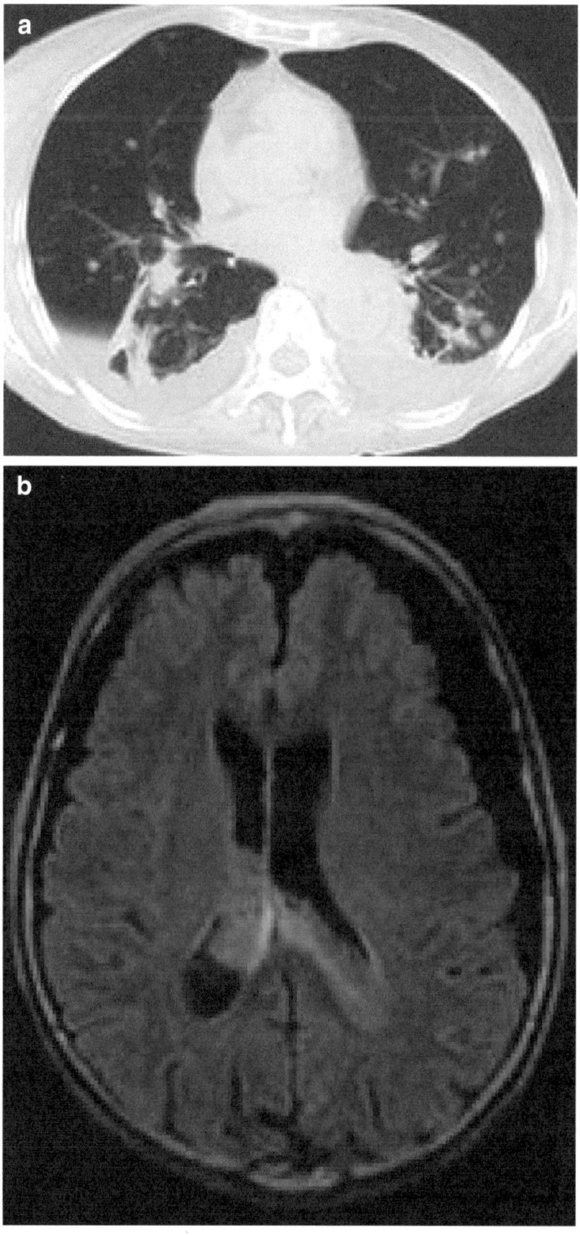

Fig. 2.3 Chest computed tomography (CT) and magnetic resonance imaging (MRI) of patients with *Scedosporium* infection. (**a**) Taken on hospital day 16, this CT scan shows bilateral smooth septal thickening, pleural effusions, multiple nodular lesions, and compressive atelectasis. (**b**) Taken on day 29 at our hospital, this MRI (axial proton-density weighted image) shows increased bilateral subdural effusion and high signal intraventricular lesions representing abscesses. Source: images from Ref. [4]

ashore and reached a shelter by herself. After being transferred to a neighboring hospital, she developed respiratory failure within a few hours of admission and was intubated under a respirator. She was transported to Iwate Medical University Hospital 5 days after drowning. Upon admission, she had a fever of 39 °C. There was no evidence of trauma or fractures anywhere on her body. Crackles were evident in both lungs. WBC was 12.9×10^9/L, and she had a neutrophilia of 11.7×10^9/L. Her serum albumin was reduced to 23 g/L, and her alkaline phosphatase was increased to 357 U/L (normal range from 99 to 340 U/L). CRP was raised to 18.5 mg/dL. CT scan of her head was normal and that of her chest revealed infiltration in both sides of her lungs (Fig. 2.4a, b). Blood culture showed no growth. A bronchoalveolar lavage (BAL) was performed. The BAL fluid contained oil, sand, and small pieces of wood (Fig. 2.5). Since Tsunami lung was suspected, treatment was started with

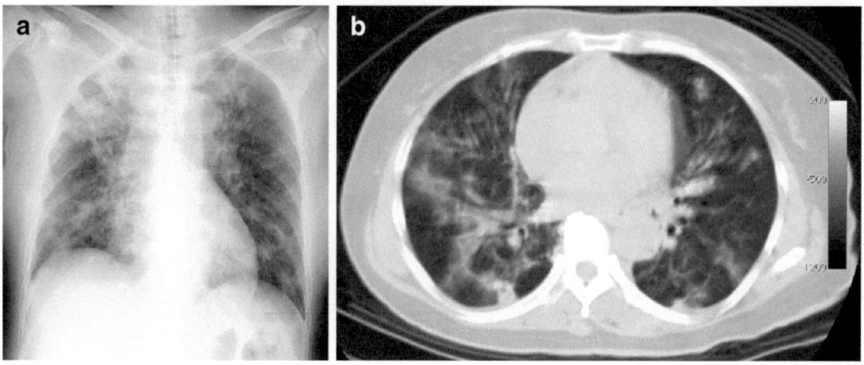

Fig. 2.4 Chest X-ray and Chest CT of a patient with Tsunami lung Case 2. (**a**) Chest X-ray of Case 2 showed bilateral infiltration without pleural effusion. (**b**) The chest CT of Case 2 showed bilateral scattered filtrates consisting alveolar filling shadows and linear infiltrations along the bronchial tree

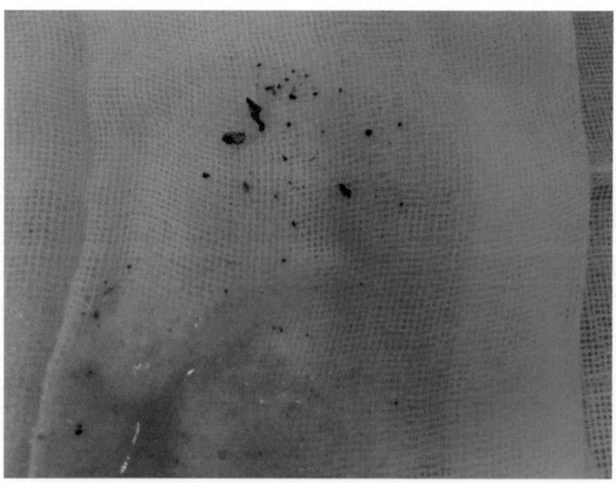

Fig. 2.5 Materials obtained from the patient with Tsunami lung by bronchoalveolar lavage. Sand particles, small pieces of woods, and bronchial mucus were observed on gauze

antibiotics, antifungal drug, and steroid pulse therapy for ARDS. Nevertheless, a follow-up CT scan of the lung on day 28 showed multiple nodular lesions of the bilateral lung and a cavity in the upper left lobe (Fig. 2.6a), and the level of βDG had increased from 11.7 to 110 pg/mL. Magnetic resonance imaging (MRI) of her head revealed multiple brain cavities (Fig. 2.6b). A new BAL was examined, and filamentous fungi, which seemed to be the cause in this case, were seen. On the basis of these results, the antimycotic therapy was switched to voriconazole.

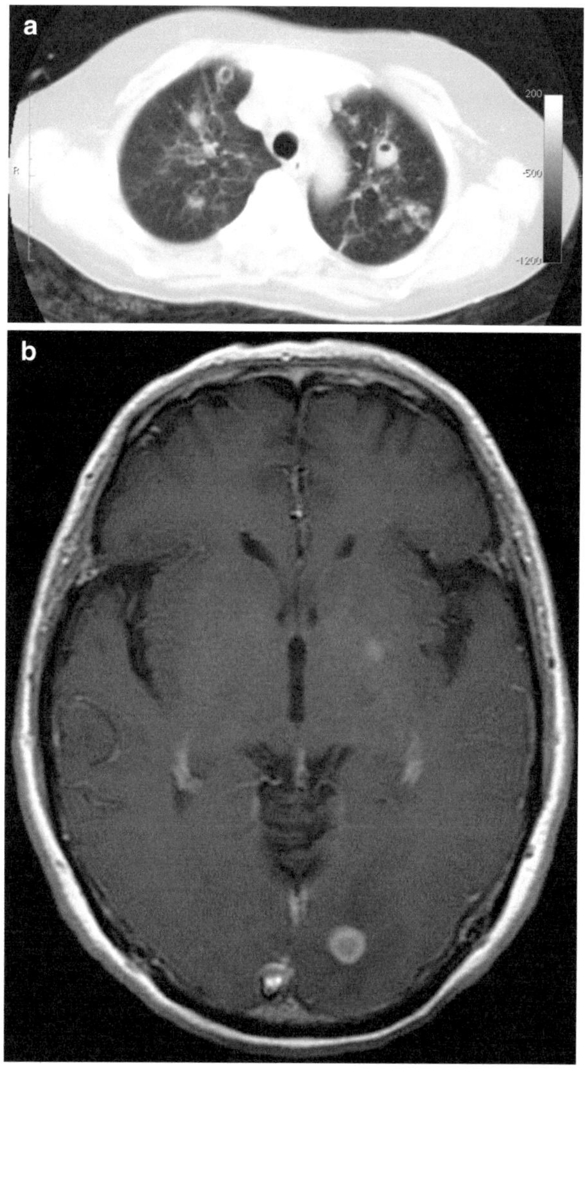

Fig. 2.6 Chest CT and brain MRI of the patient with *Scedosporium* infection. (**a**) Chest CT in Case 2 from day 28 showed a cavity in the bilateral upper lobe with a thick wall and surrounded by consolidation. (**b**) Brain MRI showed coin lesions with cavities suggesting abscesses

2.2.2.3 Case 3

A 33-year-old woman was overwhelmed by the tsunami and was rescued. Heavy oil covered her body. She was transported to the emergency center with suspicion of chemical pneumonitis. Both lungs showed diffuse infiltrative shadows on a chest X-ray. Chemical pneumonitis from aspiration of heavy oil was diagnosed. Treatment included antibiotics, sivelestat, and steroid pulse therapy.

In spite of administration of antibiotics, her respiratory state and oxygenation worsened. The chest X-ray showed alveolar infiltrates in the left upper lobe; it also showed multifocal, bilateral nodular opacities. On day 17, massive hemoptysis occurred, and the patient died because of airway occlusion.

2.2.3 Pathogen

Case 1: A diagnosis of *Scedosporium (S.) aurantiacum* infection was confirmed on day 62 at our hospital by performing polymerase chain reaction and deoxyribonucleic acid (DNA) sequencing of the filamentous fungi obtained from the BAL specimens taken on day 2 at our hospital and cultured on *Sabouraud* dextrose agar.

Case 2: Since MRI of her head on day 63 revealed multiple brain cavities, a lumbar puncture was performed but showed no white cells and no identifiable organisms on a Gram stain or upon a culture of the cerebrospinal fluid. On day 69, the diagnosis of *S. apiospermum* infection was confirmed by polymerase chain reaction and DNA sequencing of cultured filamentous fungi obtained from the first BAL specimen.

Case 3: In the BAL, *Legionella pneumophila* serogroup-1, *Pseudomonas aeruginosa*, *Stenotrophomonas maltophilia*, *Burkholderia cepacia*, and filamentous fungi *S. apiospermum* and *S. prolificans* were detected.

2.3 Discussion

Tsunami lung occurred in the patients with near-drowning who aspirated a large amount of sea water. Aspiration of sea water may cause pulmonary edema because it is 3.6% hypertonic saline and induces body fluid into alveolar spaces. In addition, the sea water in tsunami contains sand, diatom, sludge of the sea bottom, heavy oil, and microorganism. These physical, chemical, and organic insults exacerbate acute lung damages in patients with Tsunami lung. As shown in Case 2, bilateral diffuse infiltration was observed in chest X-ray, and this shadow was thought to indicate pulmonary edema. Furthermore, findings of pneumonia and alveolar hemorrhages were reported [9–12]. In the patient who aspirated large amounts of soil and sand, it was reported that increased linear intensity along with bronchi called "Sand bronchogram" was observed due to bronchi plugged with sand [13]. Because of severe respiratory failure caused by ARDS described above, steroid was often administered for treatment. It was possible that the administered steroid might provoke mycotic infection afterward.

Among the diseases caused by tsunami after Sumatra earthquake 2004, "Tsunami lung" was firstly described as a pneumonia refractory to treatment [14]. Since *Burkholderia pseudomallei* are living in soil of tropical area in Southeast Asia, pneumonia, lung abscess, and pyothorax were caused by aspiration or inhalation of muddy sea water and developed to sepsis and brain abscess as shown in the cases admitted to Iwate Medical University Hospital. *S. apiospermum* and *S. prolificans* are resident flora in soil and polluted water and may cause deep mycosis in sinus and lung via air away. Since marital generation of *S. apiospermum* was thought as *Pseudallescheria boydii* previously, they were called *pseudallescheriasis* altogether. However the two fungi are genetically different, and telemorph of *S. apiospermum* is recently identified as *Pseudallescheria apiosperma* [15].

S. apiospermum has been receiving an attention as a pathogen of opportunistic infections such as pneumonia, meningitis, osteomyelitis, sinusitis, and keratitis in patients with lowered immunocompetence by immunosuppression therapy or steroid therapy for malignant hematological diseases or organ transplantation.

Three presented cases with *scedosporiosis* admitted to Iwate Medical University hospital developed to lung abscess and brain abscess from pneumonia (Table 2.1). They were the cases of difficult-treat mycosis, finally cured by combination therapy with liposomal amphotericin and voriconazole.

S. apiospermum generally shows a high propensity to cause central nervous system (CNS) infections. The precise mechanism of *S. apiospermum* invasion and its subsequent expansion to CNS is not clarified. Probably a local spread of S. *apiospermum* from sites near the brain, such as the paranasal sinuses [16] or cribriform plate [17], may occur after a near-drowning. In addition, a hematogenous spread to CNS from the lungs is also possible. Voriconazole has been thought to be effective on CNS-related *scedosporiosis* refractory to treatment with other antifungal agents

Table 2.1 Clinical features and pathogens of patients with Tsunami lung

Case	Age/sex	Clinical manifestation	Clinical diagnosis	Pathogen	Outcome
Case 1	68/F	Fever	Pneumonia	*S. aurantiacum*	Survived
		Double hemiplegia	Brain abscess		
Case 2	59/F	Fever	Lung abscess	*S. apiospermum*	Survived
			Brain abscess		
Case 3	33/F	Respiratory failure	Pneumonia	*S. apiospermum*	Dead
		Septic shock		*S. prolificans*	
Garzoni et al. [43]	59/M	Fever, cough	Pneumonia	*S. apiospermum*	Survived
		Back pain		*P. boydii*	
Garzoni et al. [43]	51/F	Fever	Brain abscess	*S. apiospermum*	Survived
		Altered consciousness		*P. boydii*	

[18–20]. Another study described voriconazole concentrations that are higher in cerebrospinal fluid than in plasma in a female patient [21]. In case 1, voriconazole appeared to be effective but was accompanied by PVCs and was discontinued. However, in vitro susceptibility studies have shown that *S. apiospermum* isolates are susceptible to voriconazole and appear to have variable susceptibility to amphotericin B [20, 22–25]. In case 1, susceptibility testing showed that the MIC for amphotericin B was relatively low, and higher MICs were evaluated for flucytosine, fluconazole, itraconazole, miconazole, and micafungin. We added low-dose voriconazole to amphotericin B due to enhanced antifungal activity in combinations of amphotericin B plus azoles [26, 27], in vitro. The synergistic interaction on our patient can be evaluated even though low-dose voriconazole was administered.

In addition to mycotic infection in Tsunami lung, bacterial infections have been also reported. *Pseudomonas* and *Acinetobacter* were detected in the culture of sputa from patients with drowning in Sumatra-Andaman tsunami in 2004 [28, 29]. In Japan, *Pseudomonas*, *Staphylococcus aureus*, *Aspergillus flavus*, and *Aspergillus fumigatus* were detected in the culture of sputa from patients with drowning by tsunami due to the earthquake off the southwest coast of Hokkaido 1994 [30].

While a *Legionella* infection was not reported following the tsunami of the Sumatra-Andaman earthquake in 2004, there were the reports of a *Legionella* infection after the disaster of GEJET. Pathogens involved in the disease may differ according to the region. *Legionella* species inhabit freshwater environments and have been detected in rivers and brackish water areas. Patients with Legionnaires' disease in GEJET were rescued in a neighborhood near a river that was struck by the tsunami. Since community-acquired pneumonia by *Legionella pneumophila* is extremely rare in Thailand and in New Zealand and Australia, where *Legionella longbeachae* accounts for about half of Legionnaires' disease cases [31], there was difference in bacteria species in the living environment as *Legionella* bacteria multiply in man-made environmental waters.

In the patients with Tsunami lung, infections by multiple pathogens were often reported. Among tsunami victims of the Sumatra-Andaman earthquake in 2004, 7 of 16 pulmonary infection cases with microbiological examination were polymicrobial [3, 14, 32, 33]. There was a combined infection of *Legionella* and *E. coli*, and the female patient developed necrotizing pneumonia in GEJET [34].

Although a case with *Legionella pneumophila* infection after near-drowning has been reported, *Legionella* infection in a case of near-drowning in sea water or in tsunami waters has not been reported [35]. Further, inhibitory effect of sea water on the growth of *Legionella pneumophila* has been reported [36]. The patient was engulfed by the tsunami 1 km inland distant from the seashore. Thus, she might not aspirate simple sea water in Tsunami.

As described above, the cause of aspiration pneumonia seen in Tsunami lung is polymicrobial, including fungi and aerobic and anaerobic bacteria, but *Aspergillus* infection is rarely reported. Several types of infections caused by *Aspergillus* were reported in the aftermath of the 2004 Indian Ocean earthquake and tsunami [37, 38].

Despite healthy individuals, this case contracted refractory systemic *Aspergillus* infections after Tsunami lung. However, it is postulated that the patient had aspirated vast amounts of *Aspergillus* in a short time into the damaged lung during the near-drowning experience. Later, complication by disseminated aspergillosis was diagnosed during autopsy.

Concerning tuberculosis, it was reported that the annual death toll from tuberculosis in the Indian Ocean region is two to three times higher than the toll from the tsunami after Sumatra earthquake on December 26, 2004 [39]. There was no case report of Tsunami lung associated with pulmonary tuberculosis after GEJET; however retrospective study revealed that patients with tuberculosis were significantly more likely to be refugees in tsunami-affected areas [40].

Since nontuberculous mycobacteria (NTM) are ubiquitous in water and soil, there is a potential for increased exposure to these organisms during natural disasters [41]. A study conducted 4 years after Hurricane Ike and 7 years after Hurricanes Katrina and Rita reported that the relative risk of pulmonary NTM disease in residents of disaster areas was the highest in the United States [42]. The number of positive NTM sputum cultures per year in Louisiana increased in the years following these three epic hurricanes. However, there were few reports of NTM infection in GEJET. Due to the insidious nature of NTM infection, it was not likely to appear prominent as an acute or subacute infectious disease. A long-term study on NTM infection is needed after GEJET [43].

2.4 Conclusion

Clinical records of the patients with Tsunami lung in GEJET were reviewed. Tsunami lung was initiated by the aspiration of sea water including sand, sludge from the sea bottom, petroleum, and undefined chemicals. After lung damage and ARDS caused by aspirated materials, pulmonary infection with microorganisms occurred. The pneumonia in Tsunami lung caused by multiple pathogens including fungi was often refractory to treatment. *Scedosporium* species were one of the pathogens identified in patients with Tsunami lung.

Acknowledgment The authors are grateful to Mr. Brent Bell for critical reading of the manuscript.

References

1. Potera C. In disaster's wake: tsunami lung. Environ Health Perspect. 2005;113:A734.
2. Kongsaengdao S, Bunnag S, Siriwiwattnakul N. Treatment of survivors after the tsunami. N Engl J Med. 2005;352:2654–5.
3. Allworth AM. Tsunami lung: a necrotising pneumonia in survivors of the Asian tsunami. Med J Aust. 2005;182:364.
4. Nakamura Y, Suzuki N, Nakajima Y, Utsumi Y, Murata O, Nagashima H, Saito H, Sasaki N, Fujimura I, Ogino Y, Kato K, Terayama Y, Miyamoto S, Yarita K, Kamei K, Nakadate T, Endo

S, Shibuya K, Yamauchi K. *Scedosporium aurantiacum* brain abscess after near-drowning in a survivor of a tsunami in Japan. Respir Investig. 2013;51:207–11.
5. Hiruma T, Nakamura K, Inokuchi R, Kurata H, Gunshin M, Matsubara T, Ishii T, Nakajima S, Yahagi N, Shinohara K. Tsunami lung accompanied by multiple disorders. Am J Respir Crit Care Med. 2013;187:110–1.
6. Nukiwa T. An overview of respiratory medicine during the Tsunami Disaster at Tohoku, Japan, on March 11, 2011. Respir Investig. 2012;50:124–8.
7. Nakamura Y, Utsumi Y, Suzuki N, Nakajima Y, Murata O, Sasaki N, Nitanai H, Nagashima H, Miyamoto S, Yaegashi J, Hatakeyama T, Shibano Y, Yarita K, Kamei K, Nakadate T, Endo S, Terayama Y, Yamauchi K. Multiple *Scedosporium apiospermum* abscesses in a woman survivor of a tsunami in northeastern Japan: a case report. J Med Case Rep. 2011;5:526.
8. Nakadate T, Nakamura Y, Yamauchii K, Endo S. Two cases of severe pneumonia after the 2011 Great East Japan Earthquake. Western Pac Surveill Response J. 2012;3:67–70.
9. Rosenbaum HT, Thompson WL, Fuller RH. Radiographic pulmonary changes in near-drowning. Radiology. 1964;83:306–12.
10. Hasan S, Avery WG, Fabian C, Sackner MA. Near drowning in humans, a report of 36 patients. Chest. 1971;159:191–7.
11. Hunter TB, Whitehouse WM. Fresh-water near-drowning: radiological aspects. Radiology. 1974;112:51–6.
12. Putman CE, Tummillo AM, Myerson DA. Drowning: another plunge. Am J Roentgenol. 1975;125:543–8.
13. Bonilla-Santiago J, Fill WL. Sand aspiration in drowning and near drowning. Radiology. 1978;128:301–2.
14. Chierakul W, Winothai W, Wattanawaitunechai C, Wuthiekanun V, Rugtaengan T, Rattanalertnavee J, Jitpratoom P, Chaowagul W, Singhasivanon P, White NJ, Day NP, Peacock SJ. *Melioidosis* in 6 tsunami survivors in southern Thailand. Clin Infect Dis. 2005;41:982–90.
15. Gilgado F, Gené J, Cano J, Guarro J. Heterothallism in *Scedosporium apiospernum* and description of its teleomorph *Pseudallescheria apiosperma* sp. nov. Med Mycol. 2010;48:122–8.
16. Fisher JF, Shadomy S, Teabeaut JR, Woodward J, Michaels GE, Newman MA, White E, Cook P, Seagraves A, Yaghmai F, Rissing JP. Near-drowning complicated by brain abscess due to *Petriellidium boydii*. Arch Neurol. 1982;39:511–3.
17. Hachimi-Idrissi S, Willemsen M, Desprechins B, Naessens A, Goossens A, De Meirleir L, Ramet J. *Pseudallescheria boydii* and brain abscesses. Pediatr Infect Dis J. 1990;9:737–41.
18. Perfect JR, Marr KA, Walsh TJ, Greenberg RN, DuPont B, de la Torre-Cisneros J, Just-Nübling G, Schlamm HT, Lutsar I, Espinel-Ingroff A, Johnson E. Voriconazole treatment for less-common, emerging, or refractory fungal infections. Clin Infect Dis. 2003;36:1122–31.
19. Schwartz S, Reisman A, Troke PF. The efficacy of voriconazole in the treatment of 192 fungal central nervous system infections: a retrospective analysis. Infection. 2011;39:201–10.
20. Espinel-Ingroff A, Johnson E, Hockey H, Troke P. Activities of voriconazole, itraconazole and amphotericin B in vitro against 590 moulds from 323 patients in the voriconazole phase III clinical studies. J Antimicrob Chemother. 2008;61:616–20.
21. Elter T, Sieniawski M, Gossmann A, Wickenhauser C, Schröder U, Seifert H, Kuchta J, Burhenne J, Riedel KD, Fätkenheuer G, Cornely OA. Voriconazole brain tissue levels in rhinocerebral aspergillosis in a successfully treated young woman. Int J Antimicrob Agents. 2006;28:262–5.
22. Meletiadis J, Meis JF, Mouton JW, Rodriquez-Tudela JL, Donnelly JP, Verweij PE. EUROFUNG Network: *in vitro* activities of new and conventional antifungal agents against clinical *Scedosporium* isolates. Antimicrob Agents Chemother. 2002;46:62–8.
23. Cuenca-Estrella M, Gomez-Lopez A, Mellado E, Buitrago MJ, Monzon A, Rodriguez-Tudela JL. Head-to-head comparison of the activities of currently available antifungal agents against 3,378 Spanish clinical isolates of yeasts and filamentous fungi. Antimicrob Agents Chemother. 2006;50:917–21.
24. Katragkou A, Dotis J, Kotsiou M, Tamiolaki M, Roilides E. *Scedosporium apiospermum* infection after near-drowning. Mycoses. 2007;50:412–21.

25. Troke P, Aguirrebengoa K, Arteaga C, Ellis D, Heath CH, Lutsar I, Rovira M, Nguyen Q, Slavin M, Chen SC. Global Scedosporium Study Group: treatment of *Scedosporiosis* with voriconazole: clinical experience with 107 patients. Antimicrob Agents Chemother. 2008;52:1743–50.
26. Walsh TJ, Peter J, McGough DA, Fothergill AW, Rinaldi MG, Pizzo PA. Activities of amphotericin B and antifungal azoles alone and in combination against *Pseudallescheria boydii*. Antimicrob Agents Chemother. 1995;39:1361–4.
27. Rodríguez MM, Calvo E, Serena C, Mariné M, Pastor FJ, Guarro J. Effects of double and triple combinations of antifungal drugs in a murine model of disseminated infection by *Scedosporium prolificans*. Antimicrob Agents Chemother. 2009;53:2153–5.
28. Kateruttanakul P, Paovilai W, Kongsaengdao S, Bunnag S, Atipornwanich K, Siriwatanakul N. Respiratory complication of tsunami victims in Phuket and Phang Nga. J Med Assoc Thail. 2005;88:754–8.
29. Yorsaengrat W, Chungpaibulpatana J, Tunki B, Pauvilai W, Kititornkul S, Suntong B. Respiratory complication of tsunami disaster victims in Vachira Phuket Hospital. J Med Assoc Thail. 2006;89:518–21.
30. Hoshino H, Watanabe H, Saitoh Y, Shibuya Y, Koba H, Abe S. A case of sea water and sand aspiration during near drowning. J Jpn Respir Soc. 1998;36:306–10. (in Japanese)
31. Phares CR, Wangroongsarb P, Chantra S, Paveenkitiporn W, Tondella ML, Benson RF, Thacker WL, Fields BS, Moore MR, Fischer J, Dowell SF, Olsen SJ. Epidemiology of severe pneumonia caused by *Legionella longbeachae*, *Mycoplasma pneumoniae*, and *Chlamydia pneumoniae*: 1-year, population-based surveillance for severe pneumonia in Thailand. Clin Infect Dis. 2007;45:e147–55.
32. Athan E, Allworth AM, Engler C, Bastian I, Cheng AC. *Melioidosis* in tsunami survivors. Emerg Infect Dis. 2005;11:1638–9.
33. Othman N, Ismail IH, Yip R, Zainuddin Z, Kasim SM, Isa R, Noh LM. Infections in post-tsunami victims. Pediatr Infect Dis J. 2007;26:960–1.
34. Ebisawa K, Yamada N, Okada S, Suzuki Y, Satoh A, Kobayashi M, Morikawa N. Combined *Legionella* and *Escherichia coli* lung infection after a tsunami disaster. Intern Med. 2011;50:2233–6.
35. Shiota R, Takeshita K, Yamamoto K, Imada K, Yabuuchi E, Wang L. *Legionella pneumophila* serogroup 3 isolated from a patient of pneumonia developed after drowning in bathtub of a hot spring spa. Kansenshogaku Zasshi. 1995;69:1356–64. (in Japanese, Abstract in English)
36. Tsuchiya Y, Terao M, Fujimoto T, Nakamura K, Yamamoto M. Effects of Japan Sea proper water on the growth of *Legionella pneumophila*, *Escherichia coli*, and *Staphylococcus aureus*. Environ Health Prev Med. 2005;10:233–8.
37. Kao AY, Munandar R, Ferrara SL, Systrom DM, Sheridan RL, Cash SS, Ryan ET. Case records of the Massachusetts General Hospital. Case 19-2005. A 17-year-old girl with respiratory distress and hemiparesis after surviving a tsunami. N Engl J Med. 2005;352:2628–36.
38. Gunaratne PS, Wijeyaratne CN, Seneviratne HR. *Aspergillus* meningitis in Sri Lanka - a post-tsunami effect? N Engl J Med. 2007;356:754–6.
39. Bastian I. The tsunami of tuberculosis. Med J Aust. 2005;182:263–4.
40. Kanamori H, Hatakeyama T, Uchiyama B, Weber DJ, Takeuchi M, Endo S, Hirakata Y, Kaku M. Clinical and molecular epidemiological features of tuberculosis after the 2011 Japan earthquake and tsunami. Int J Tuberc Lung Dis. 2016;20:505–14.
41. Honda JR, Bernhard JN, Chan ED. Natural disasters and nontuberculous mycobacteria: a recipe for increased disease? Chest. 2015;147:304–8.
42. Adjemian J, Olivier KN, Seitz AE, Falkinham JO III, Holland SM, Prevots DR. Spatial clusters of nontuberculous mycobacterial lung disease in the United States. Am J Respir Crit Care Med. 2012;186:553–8.
43. Garzoni C, Emonet S, Legout L, Benedict R, Hoffmeyer P, Bernard L, Garbino J. Atypical infections in Tsunami survivors. Emerg Infect Dis. 2005;11:1591–3.

Chapter 3
Respiratory Tract Burns, Traumatic Pulmonary Contusions, Crushing Death, and Crush Syndrome: What Kinds of Lung Injury Occur by Respiratory Tract Burn, Traumatic Contusion, and Crush Syndrome?

Hiroshi Imamura

Abstract Various types of respiratory system injury can occur in a disaster setting, including traumatic thoracic injury, traumatic asphyxia, and inhalation injury. Further, multi-system injuries may occur in combination with those affecting the respiratory system. Acute respiratory distress syndrome often complicates disaster-related injuries, such as crush syndrome, thoracic trauma, hemorrhagic shock, and burns. Poor hygiene, air and water pollution, malnutrition arising from food shortages, and shortages of medical resources in a disaster setting can aggravate the course of a disaster-related injury. A large number of casualties may occur at the scene of a disaster. The principle in disaster medicine is to provide the best treatment to the greatest number of victims using limited medical resources. Treatment of patients with severe injuries or complicated needs consumes a considerable amount of these resources. Therefore, victims should be transported to facilities outside the disaster zone as soon as possible for further treatment after vital signs are stabilized.

Keywords Inhalation injury · Thoracic trauma · Pulmonary contusion · Asphyxia · Crush syndrome

---

H. Imamura
Department of Emergency and Critical Care Medicine, Shinshu University School of Medicine, Matsumoto, Japan
e-mail: imamura@shinshu-u.ac.jp

K. Fujimoto (ed.), *Disaster and Respiratory Diseases*,
Respiratory Disease Series: Diagnostic Tools and Disease Managements,
https://doi.org/10.1007/978-981-13-2598-4_3

3.1 Introduction

Various types of respiratory system injuries can occur at the time of a disaster. In the event of natural disasters, such as earthquakes or volcanic eruptions, both traumatic and inhalation injuries may occur when a building collapses or catches fire. Tropical storms, floods, landslides, and tornadoes often cause traumatic lung injuries, as does drowning or near-drowning. Man-made disasters, such as those involving transport and use of weapons of mass destruction, also cause inhalation and traumatic injuries, including blast lung injuries. This chapter discusses inhalation injuries, traumatic injuries of the respiratory system, and crush injuries.

3.2 Inhalation Injury

There may be many patients with burns and inhalation injuries at the scene of a fire-related disaster. During the last three decades, the prognosis of patients with major thermal injury has improved significantly with advances in the overall care of burns patients. However, inhalation injury significantly increases mortality [1]. Half of all fire-related deaths are attributable to smoke inhalation. Further, there are a number of impediments to efficient care in disaster settings, including delayed rescue and transport services, poor access to medical supplies, poor initial assessment by physicians inexperienced in treating burns patients, and a shortage of medical resources. Even a patient with major burns may not have a high degree of urgency, but a patient with inhalation injury can deteriorate rapidly because of airway compromise and can be a true emergency.

3.2.1 Pathophysiology

Inhalation injury is caused by exposure to heat and inhalation of toxic products of incomplete combustion and particulate matter. Inhalation injuries are classified as thermal injuries to the upper airways, chemical irritation and injuries to the respiratory tract, and systemic toxicity upon exposure to noxious gases [2–4].

Thermal injury usually affects the upper airways. Thermal injury below the vocal cords is uncommon because of the highly efficient heat exchange system in the pharynx and the reflex mechanism of laryngeal closure. Steam has 400 times the heat-carrying capacity of dry heat and can cause lower airway injury. Like burns of the skin, thermal injury in the airways damages epithelial cells, denatures proteins, and initiates a cascade of inflammatory responses. These responses result in formation of edema in the epiglottis and swelling of the tongue, causing airway obstruction.

Small particles may reach the terminal bronchioles, where they can initiate an inflammatory reaction leading to bronchospasm and edema. Chemical irritants also damage epithelial cells in the airway, producing mucosal edema of the small airways and decreasing the activity of alveolar surfactants, leading to bronchospasm, airflow obstruction, atelectasis, and pulmonary edema. Acute respiratory distress syndrome (ARDS) may also develop. With time, tracheal and bronchial epithelial sloughing occurs.

Toxic gases are divided into three broad groups, i.e., pulmonary irritants, tissue asphyxiants, and systemic toxins. The two major tissue asphyxiants are carbon monoxide and hydrogen cyanide. Carbon monoxide has an affinity for hemoglobin that is 200 times higher than its affinity for oxygen. Severe carbon monoxide poisoning causes hypoxia in the brain and disturbance of consciousness. Cyanides are formed when nitrogen-containing polymers are burned. Cyanides bind to the mitochondria, where they disrupt oxidative phosphorylation, leading to profound tissue hypoxia.

3.2.2 Clinical Features

The diagnosis of inhalation injury can be highly subjective and is made from the history of a fire in an enclosed space and physical signs that include facial burns, singed nasal hair, soot in the mouth or nose, hoarseness, carbonaceous sputum, and expiratory wheeze (Fig. 3.1). Upper airway edema can occur rapidly, but lower airway edema is usually not clinically evident for up to 24 h.

3.2.3 Prehospital Care and Emergency Management

A 100% oxygen mask should be applied from the scene of the injury to the hospital because of possible carbon monoxide poisoning. General and dermal care for burns patients will be described elsewhere.

Initial assessment of a patient with burns is divided into a primary survey and a secondary survey [5]. In the primary survey, the ABCs should be assessed and stabilized. Airway management is especially important. It is possible for the airway to swell rapidly, even though the patient can speak and has no dyspnea initially. The patient should be examined for signs of inhalation injury, evidence of facial burns, carbonaceous sputum, singed nasal hair, and soot in the mouth. If there is any evidence of airway compromise accompanied by swelling of the neck, burns inside the mouth, or wheezing, tracheal intubation should be performed.

In the secondary survey, a directed history should be obtained from the patient and emergency medical service personnel. These include exposure to a burning

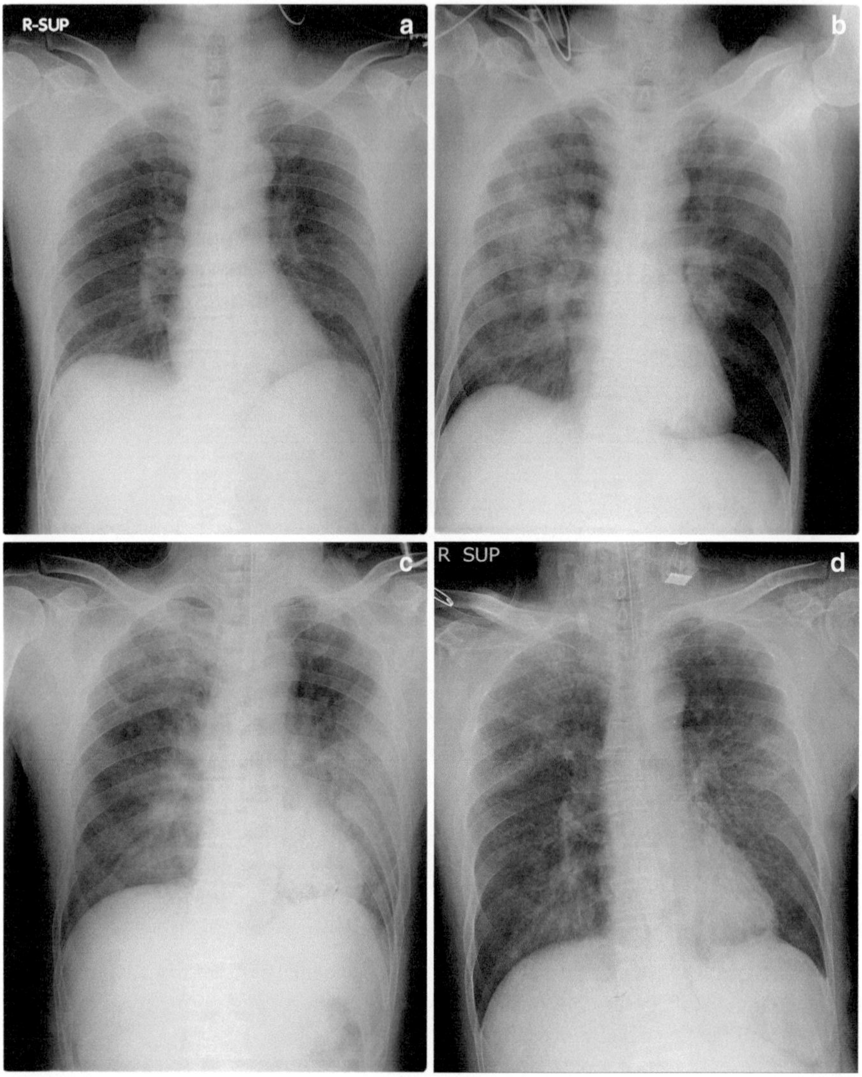

Fig. 3.1 Inhalation injury in a patient who was transferred to hospital after extinguishing a house fire. On admission, he had cough but did not have any hoarseness, stridor, wheeze, or evidence of facial burns. A chest radiograph (**a**) revealed no abnormality. Fiber-optic bronchoscopy showed a little soot but no edema or erythema in the larynx. The patient had dyspnea on day 2 (chest radiograph, **b**). A diagnosis of smoke inhalation injury without thermal injury was made. The patient was intubated on day 3 (chest radiograph, **c**). Chest computed tomography on the same day (**f**) showed bilateral infiltrative shadowing, ground-glass opacities, and bronchial stenoses. Fiber-optic bronchoscopy on day 3 (**g**), day 5 (**h**), and day 6 (**i**) revealed mucosal edema, sloughing of necrotic endobronchial debris, and complete denudation of the bronchial mucosa, respectively. The infiltrative shadowing seen on the chest radiograph started to resolve on day 5 (**d**). However, frequent bronchoscopy was needed to remove debris and airway casts thereafter. Fiber-optic bronchoscopy on day 12 (**j**) showed healing of the bronchial mucosal injury. The patient was successfully extubated on day 15. A chest radiograph on day 19 (**e**) showed the lungs were clear, except for an old inflammatory lesion in the left middle lung field

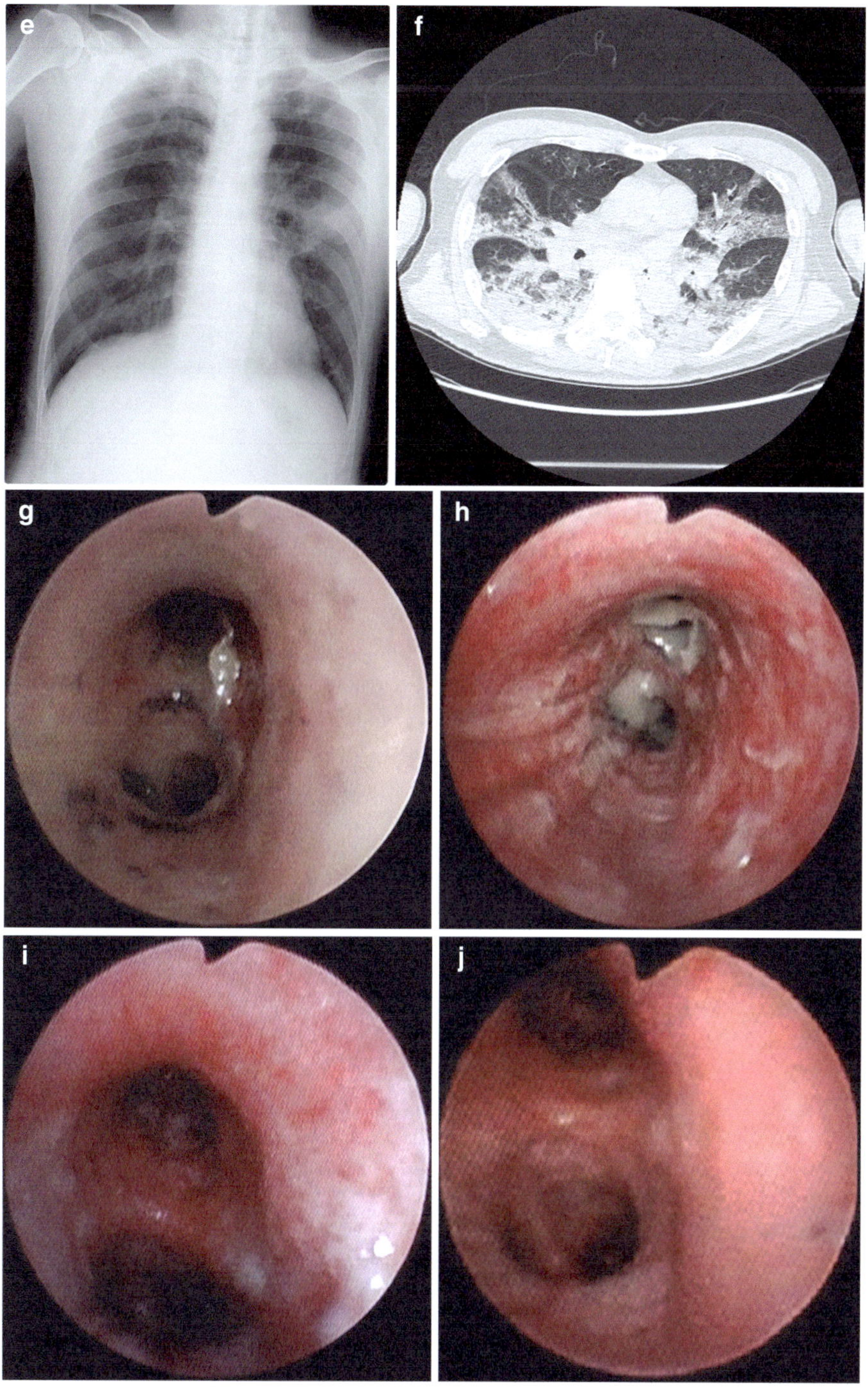

Fig. 3.1 (continued)

agent, involvement of chemicals, duration of exposure, exposure to fire in an open or enclosed space, presence or absence of an explosion, other trauma, and loss of consciousness. Arterial blood gases, including a carboxyhemoglobin level, a chest radiograph, and an electrocardiogram, should be obtained. If there is any doubt regarding the presence of airway edema or inhalation injury, fiber-optic bronchoscopy or direct laryngoscopy should be performed using topical anesthesia. If the airway appears normal, tracheal intubation may be deferred. However, such patients may still require close observation or repeat evaluation of the airway if conditions change. Early tracheal intubation should be strongly considered in patients with extensive burns (i.e., involving >40% of the total body surface area) in the absence of inhalation injury because formation of edema may progress to impairment or occlusion of the airway within minutes to hours. If tracheal intubation is indicated, this should be performed using topical anesthesia with the patient awake, although moderate sedation is recommended. Tracheal intubation under the guidance of fiber-optic bronchoscopy may be required. Routine "prophylactic" tracheal intubation may be harmful in many patients.

3.2.4 Treatment in the Intensive Care Unit

Treatment of inhalation injury includes humidified oxygen, intubation and ventilation, bronchodilators, and pulmonary toilet. Bronchoscopy in the subacute stage may reveal necrosis of the tracheobronchial mucosa and hemorrhagic tracheobronchitis. At this stage, therapeutic bronchoscopy should be performed to relieve airway obstruction caused by necrotic debris in the tracheobronchial tree [6]. It should be noted that ventilator-associated lung injury plays a role in the ARDS often seen in patients with presumed inhalation injury [7]. Half of patients with inhalation injury will develop pulmonary infection [6]. Any patient who has fever and purulent sputum should be treated with antibiotics guided by sputum culture. Pulmonary toilet is especially important.

Circulatory (hypovolemic as well as distributive) shock often occurs in patients with moderate to major burns. The Baxter or Parkland formula is usually used to guide burn shock fluid resuscitation [8]. Inhalation injury has been shown to increase total fluid needs. About half of intubated burns patients develop ARDS. Therefore, when inhalation injury is present, fluid resuscitation should be performed carefully to avoid exacerbating pulmonary edema and ARDS [3]. Patients with moderate to major burns need prolonged respiratory support.

Treatment of a patient with major burns involves intensive care over a long period of time and consumes a large amount of medical resources. Unlike a patient with trauma, a patient with major burns generally does not have a high degree of urgency if the airway is ensured. Thus, patients with moderate to major burns should be transported to facilities outside the disaster zone within 24 h [6].

3.3 Thoracic Trauma: General Principles and Initial Management

3.3.1 General Principles

Thoracic trauma is responsible for 20–25% of all trauma deaths and is second only to head trauma as the primary cause of death at injury scenes [9]. Many thoracic trauma deaths occur soon after the patient reaches the hospital. In-hospital mortality is reported to be low (5%) for isolated chest injuries but increases to 37% in patients with injuries involving multiple organ systems [10]. The mortality rate can increase significantly if initial treatment is delayed or medical resources are poor at the scene of a disaster. Of note, minor injuries, such as a simple rib fracture, can cause significant morbidity and mortality if initial treatment is inadequate, hygiene is inadequate, and the environment at the scene of the disaster is poor.

When managing mass casualties in disaster settings, patients with severe injuries should be transported to facilities outside the disaster zone for definitive treatment or intensive care after initial stabilization. Patients with thoracic trauma may develop unstable hemodynamic or respiratory states. Progression of underlying injuries, inadequacy of care during transport, and the physical stress of transport can lead to clinical deterioration of the patient en route to hospital. A high-quality critical care transport team is needed. Further, the risks and benefits of transport should be considered.

Injuries of the tracheobronchial tree, heart, esophagus, thoracic great vessels, and penetrating thoracic injuries are described in detail elsewhere [11].

3.3.2 Initial Management

Patients with chest trauma and severe respiratory distress have a high mortality rate [11]. It should be borne in mind that the cause of respiratory distress is not always an injury involving the respiratory system. The most frequent causes of respiratory distress are shock, coma, multiple rib fractures, and hemopneumothorax. Diagnosis of the cause of respiratory distress must be made promptly. If the patient is making little or no effort to breathe, central nervous system dysfunction as a result of head trauma or spinal cord injury is the most likely cause. If the patient is attempting to breathe but is moving little or no air, upper airway obstruction caused by the tongue base falling backward, dislodged dentures, vomitus, or blood clots should be suspected. Traumatic fracture of the larynx or trachea can cause airway obstruction. If the upper airway appears intact but the breath sounds are poor, thoracic problems such as flail chest, hemopneumothorax, diaphragmatic injury, or parenchymal lung damage should be considered.

In all cases of respiratory distress, the airway must be secured. A surgical cricothyroidotomy should be performed promptly if tracheal intubation is difficult. When the airway is controlled, optimal oxygenation and ventilation should be provided.

One of the most common times for a patient to have a cardiac arrest in the emergency department is during or immediately after tracheal intubation [3, 11]. Common causes of cardiac arrest during intubation include esophageal intubation and inadequate oxygenation pre-intubation. Physicians should recognize that cardiac arrest can occur even after technically correct tracheal intubation because of reduced venous return, tension pneumothorax, systemic air embolism, or a sudden decrease in sympathetic tone.

3.4 Thoracic Trauma: Injury to the Chest Wall

3.4.1 Simple Rib Fractures

3.4.1.1 Clinical Features

Rib fractures are common injuries [12]. Traumatic rib fractures occur most often at the site of direct impact or at the posterolateral angle, which is structurally the weakest area of the thoracic cage. The most frequent symptom of a rib fracture is pain. Patients can often localize the pain to one or two ribs and can reproduce or exacerbate the pain by taking a deep breath. Fractures of the first, second, or third ribs indicate a high-energy mechanism and may be associated with major vascular injuries. Fractures of the ninth, tenth, or eleventh ribs sometimes cause injuries to intra-abdominal organs, such as the liver or spleen. Physicians should have a low threshold of suspicion for rib fractures in patients with blunt chest trauma because up to 50% of fractures may be undetected radiographically [13].

3.4.1.2 Treatment

Rib fractures can be very painful, causing decreased chest wall excursion/respiratory splitting that results in atelectasis, pneumonia, and possibly hypoxemia. Thus, the major goal in the management of rib fractures is pain control and identification of patients who are likely to develop complications. The pain should be relieved early and adequately. Nonsteroidal anti-inflammatory drugs with or without opioids are generally prescribed for mild to moderate chest wall pain. For more severe injuries, particularly if ventilation is compromised and the patient has been admitted, an intercostal nerve block may be needed. Epidural anesthesia usually works better, but monitoring for apnea is needed. Rib belts are not recommended because they compromise ventilatory function and should be considered only for young patients with few rib fractures.

3.4.1.3 Special Consideration for Elderly Patients

Elderly patients are at increased risk of complications from rib fractures. One overview of 77 elderly patients reported that an isolated rib fracture was associated with a 38% rate of respiratory complications and a mortality rate of 8% [14]. Comorbid conditions also play an important role in the risks of intubation and pneumonia following rib fractures in elderly patients. These include chronic obstructive pulmonary disease, protein-calorie malnutrition, need for an ambulatory assist device, congestive heart failure, spinal fracture, and lower limb fractures. These comorbidities are often aggravated by poor environmental hygiene or malnutrition. Physicians should be aware that elderly patients with even simple rib fractures could develop severe complications in a disaster setting.

3.4.2 Flail Chest

3.4.2.1 Clinical Features

The most severe form of blunt thoracic wall skeletal injury is a flail chest, defined as two or more fractures in three or more contiguous ribs. This injury results in paradoxical inward movement of a segment of the chest wall during spontaneous inspiration and outward movement during expiration. The paradoxical motion of the chest wall greatly increases the work of breathing or respiratory effort. Underlying pulmonary contusion may cause severe hypoxemia. Such patients have dyspnea, ventilator fatigue, and hypoxia.

3.4.2.2 Treatment

Pain control and adequate ventilation are crucial to prevent respiratory failure in these patients [13]. Patients with mild to moderate flail chest and no underlying pulmonary contusion can often be managed without a ventilator. Adequate pain relief using oral analgesics, regional nerve block, or epidural anesthesia is needed, along with chest physiotherapy to remove respiratory tract secretions. A trial of noninvasive positive pressure ventilation (NPPV) may facilitate breathing by overcoming the need to create negative pressure during inspiration. A lack of improvement in ventilatory function is an indication for tracheal intubation and mechanical ventilation. The mortality rate is extremely high if ventilator assistance is delayed until there is clinical evidence of respiratory failure. Circulatory shock, three or more associated injuries, and severe head injury are also indications for early intubation. These patients have poor ventilatory effort, so are at high risk of complications such as atelectasis and pneumonia and require further chest physiotherapy. In severe cases of flail chest, surgical fixation may be indicated, although this procedure is rarely needed.

3.5 Thoracic Trauma: Injury to the Lungs

3.5.1 Pulmonary Contusion

3.5.1.1 Pathophysiology

Pulmonary contusion occurs in most patients who sustain blunt chest trauma [3, 4, 12, 15]. The most typical cause of pulmonary contusion is a compression-decompression injury to the chest. The main pathophysiologic changes are hemorrhage and surrounding edema. The pathologic changes associated with pulmonary contusion seem to be primarily the result of capillary damage. Intra-alveolar hemorrhage occurs initially and is followed by edema. Accumulation of debris and mucus secretions causes further atelectasis, which leads to large areas of unventilated but perfused lung. Intrapulmonary shunt and resistance to airflow are increased, and lung compliance is reduced, with an increase in ventilation/perfusion mismatch. Pulmonary contusions also result in acute local and systemic inflammatory cascades that activate tissue macrophages and production of inflammatory mediators, cytokines, and chemokines. In disasters such as earthquakes, these processes are also influenced by inhalation of dust and sludge or thermal injury. The clinical result is hypoxia and increased work of breathing. Further, resuscitative measures directed at associated injuries, especially administration of intravenous fluids, cause pulmonary edema and are harmful to the lung.

3.5.1.2 Clinical Features

The clinical manifestations associated with pulmonary contusion are variable, ranging from mild dyspnea to ARDS. Some patients have bloody sputum. Pulmonary contusion may not appear on initial chest radiographs, although they are usually seen as areas of opacification of the lung by 6 h after the injury. Chest computed tomography (CT) is more sensitive for diagnosing early pulmonary contusions (Fig. 3.2). It should be noted that underlying pulmonary disease, especially chronic obstructive pulmonary disease, significantly and adversely influences the course of pulmonary contusion.

3.5.1.3 Treatment

Treatment of pulmonary contusion is supportive and includes supplemental oxygen, adequate pain control, aggressive pulmonary toilet, and judicious fluid management [15]. There is no role for either routine antibiotics or steroid therapy. Intubation and mechanical ventilation are employed only as necessary. The degree of pulmonary dysfunction usually peaks at 72 h and generally resolves within 7 days in the absence of associated nosocomial pneumonia. The major goal in the treatment of pulmonary

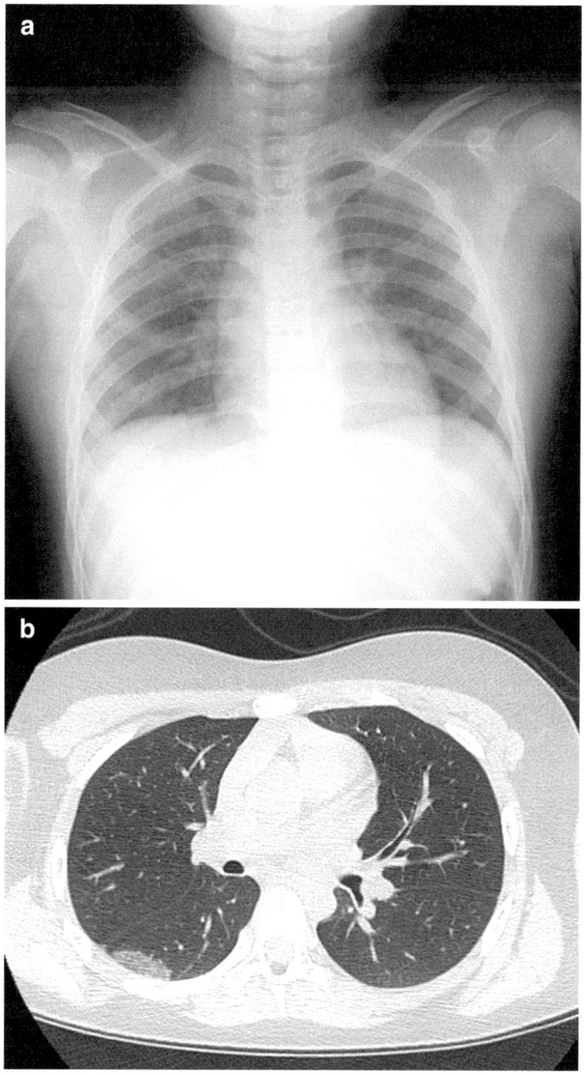

Fig. 3.2 Mild pulmonary contusion in a patient with no chest symptoms. A chest radiograph (**a**) showed no apparent abnormality. Chest computed tomography showed a small ground-glass opacity in the right lower lobe (**b**)

contusion is prevention of complications such as pneumonia, atelectasis, and ventilator-induced lung injury while waiting for the contused lungs to heal.

NPPV can be used in a selected group of patients with pulmonary contusion and hypoxemia who are refractory to supplemental oxygen. NPPV should be used in patients who are able to protect their own airway and do not have any contraindications to NPPV, such as inability to tolerate the mask, inability to cooperate, hemodynamic instability, facial injuries, or inability to cough or remove their own secretions.

Some patients with pulmonary contusion develop ARDS and pneumonia, especially if elderly. ARDS is seen particularly in the first 24–48 h after the injury.

The goal should be to re-expand atelectatic regions in a contused lung using high positive end-expiratory pressure and recruitment maneuvers. The ideal ventilation strategy follows those for ARDS [16]. Supportive therapy for ARDS is focused on limiting further ventilator-associated lung injury by lung-protective ventilation. Supportive measures include the following: a low tidal volume, at 6–8 mL/kg of predicted body weight; limited plateau pressure <30 mmHg, which is associated with less tidal hyperinflation and end-tidal collapse; a fraction of inspired oxygen that is as low as possible; and optimal positive end-expiratory pressure, incrementally added to optimize oxygenation. Provided that the pH is >7.2, elevated partial pressure of carbon dioxide levels can be tolerated if inadequate ventilation is not possible.

In patients with severe ARDS caused by pulmonary contusion, ordinary mechanical ventilation may be insufficient to maintain oxygenation. The first maneuver should be to place the uninjured lung down by turning the patient to the decubitus position. This simple maneuver can improve ventilation/perfusion mismatch. Ventilation while the patient is in the prone position is currently recommended, although some trauma patients cannot tolerate prone positioning because of injuries to other parts of the body. Successful use of high-frequency oscillatory ventilation or inhalation of nitric oxide in patients with severe pulmonary contusions has been reported [17] (Fig. 3.3). Extracorporeal membrane oxygenation can be effective for very severe ARDS if adequate lung-protective strategies fail to maintain oxygenation [18]. However, in many trauma patients, extracorporeal membrane oxygenation cannot be used because of hemorrhagic complications.

3.6 Pneumothorax and Hemothorax

3.6.1 Pneumothorax

3.6.1.1 Clinical Features

Pneumothorax is common in thoracic trauma [3]. Disruption of the visceral pleura as a result of blunt shearing or lacerations from fractured ribs allows leakage of air from the lung into the pleural space, leading to negative intrapleural pressure during inspiration. Sometimes, penetrating trauma causes air to enter the pleural space through the thoracic wall (open pneumothorax). The clinical manifestations of a pneumothorax are variable and depend on the degree of lung collapse. Symptomatology is not helpful whether the patient has a pneumothorax because many patients with thoracic trauma complain of chest pain. The decrease in vital capacity causes varying degrees of hypoxemia. If the pneumothorax is large, it can have profound effects on intrathoracic pressure, causing a mediastinal shift and hemodynamic instability by a decrease in preload and marked reduction in diastolic filling of the heart. Tension pneumothorax (Fig. 3.4) is life-threatening and manifests clinically as hypotension, elevated jugular venous pressure, hypoxemia, and dyspnea and may progress to cardiac arrest.

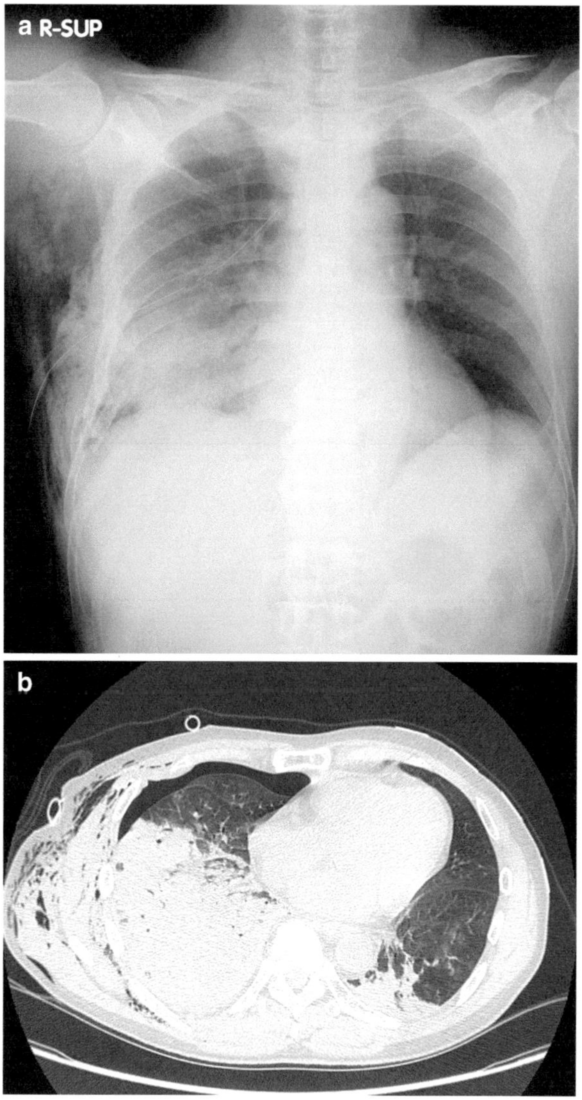

Fig. 3.3 Severe pulmonary contusion in a patient who had fallen from a roof and was transferred to hospital by ambulance. Upon arrival in the emergency room, the trachea was intubated, and a chest tube was inserted because of right tension pneumothorax. A chest radiograph (**a**) showed diffuse shadowing in the right middle and lower lung, multiple rib fractures, and subcutaneous emphysema. Chest computed tomography (**b**) revealed severe pulmonary contusion. The patient also had a hepatic injury, a right renal injury, and a pelvic fracture. He underwent separation lung ventilation because of right pulmonary hemorrhage and high-frequency oscillation ventilation thereafter and was successfully extubated on day 14

The diagnosis of pneumothorax is made on a chest radiograph or chest CT. With the growing use of CT in the management of trauma patients, small pneumothoraces that cannot be seen on a plain radiograph are often discovered (so-called occult pneumothorax). In recent years, ultrasonography has been used increasingly in the emergency department or at the scene of injury to determine whether a pneumothorax is present. Ultrasonography has been reported to be more sensitive than supine chest radiography for identifying pneumothorax. Ultrasonographic examination of the lung can be useful for detecting pneumothorax in a disaster setting.

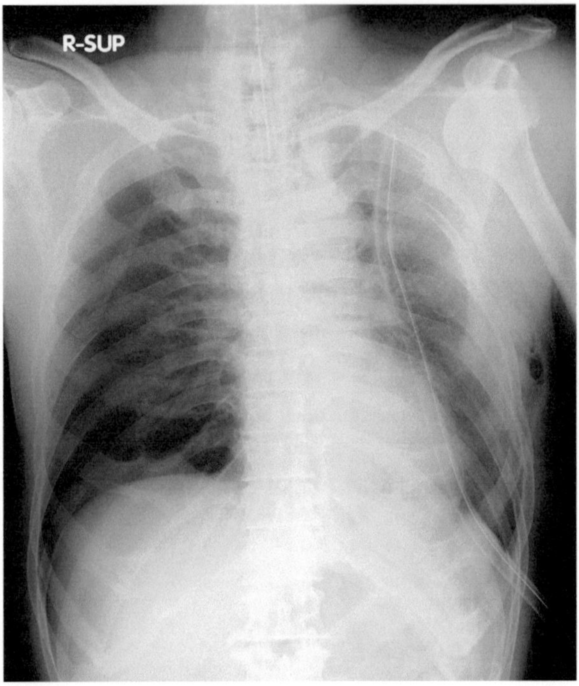

Fig. 3.4 Traumatic pneumothorax in a patient who developed shock after falling from a ladder. At the scene, the trachea was intubated, and a chest tube was inserted in the left pleural space because of bilateral tension pneumothorax. His blood pressure increased. A chest radiograph on admission showed a right pneumothorax, multiple left rib fractures, subcutaneous emphysema, and dislocation of the left shoulder joint. His left pneumothorax had improved

3.6.1.2 Treatment

Tube thoracostomy is the definitive treatment for most cases of pneumothorax. The optimal position is posterior, to facilitate dependent drainage of blood, and directed to the apex of the pleural cavity.

In cases of tension pneumothorax, immediate decompression with a large-bore needle is indicated. Many patients will require tube thoracostomy after needle decompression. Finger (simple) thoracostomy can be considered in an unstable patient, especially in a disaster setting. An incision is made in the fifth intercostal space in the lateral chest wall, and forceps are used to enter the pleural space. If a rush of air or release of hemothorax occurs, the procedure can be completed as a tube thoracostomy. Finger thoracostomy can often be performed just as rapidly as needle decompression, but with a much higher success rate.

Although large-bore tubes are typically chosen in the emergency department, the tube size can be individualized. Large tube diameters are limited by the intercostal space, so a larger tube may produce more pain without providing any additional drainage [12]. Pneumothorax and air leaks should be resolved before removal of the tube; ideally, drainage should be less than 2 mL/kg/day. After 12–24 h without an air leak, the tube may be removed while on suction.

The treatment of so-called “occult” pneumothorax is not as well defined as that for usual pneumothorax. Generally, this type of pneumothorax does not require treatment but should be monitored for progression. Prophylactic tube thoracostomy is usually performed in the setting of positive-pressure ventilation because progression to tension pneumothorax occurs in approximately 10% of patients [4].

3.6.2 Hemothorax

3.6.2.1 Clinical Features

Hemothorax is the presence of blood in the pleural space (Fig. 3.5). In addition to air, blood can also enter the pleural space secondary to thoracic trauma. Bleeding occurs most frequently from the lung parenchyma; other origins of blood include the muscles and bones of chest wall, the intercostal or internal mammary arteries, and the great vessels of the chest. A large hemothorax restricts ventilation and venous return. It should be emphasized that the hemothorax may not be apparent on an initial chest radiograph, especially if obtained with the patient in the supine position. Ultrasonography is valuable for establishing the diagnosis of hemothorax. It should be kept in mind that delayed hemothorax is not uncommon.

3.6.2.2 Treatment

Hemothorax should generally be drained by tube thoracostomy [11]. Bleeding from multiple intrathoracic vessels often ceases fairly rapidly after the hemothorax is completely evacuated. The compressing effect of the shed blood and the low pulmonary arterial pressure combine to help reduce bleeding from the lung parenchyma. Thus, a thoracotomy is not usually needed in patients with thoracic trauma. A massive hemothorax is usually the result of a major vessel injury and is life-threatening. Indications for thoracotomy include immediate return of 1500 mL of blood via tube

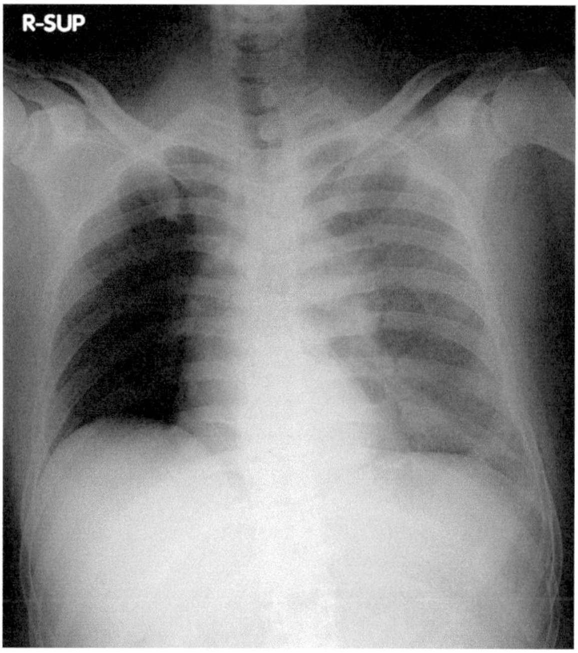

Fig. 3.5 Hemothorax in a patient who had slipped and fallen down the side of a mountain. A chest radiograph on admission showed left hemothorax and multiple rib fractures. Eight hundred milliliters of blood was drained from the thoracostomy tube

thoracostomy or continued output of more than 200 mL/h for 2–4 consecutive hours. Inadequately drained hemothorax can lead to complications, including clotted hemothorax and empyema. As with occult pneumothorax, hemothorax that is asymptomatic and found only on CT scan can be managed conservatively.

3.7 Crushing Death and Crush Syndrome

3.7.1 Crushing Death and Traumatic Asphyxia

It is reported that up to 80% of crush victims die as a result of severe head injuries or asphyxiation, with only 20% reaching hospital [19]. Sudden, severe crushing of the chest sometimes causes traumatic asphyxia [3] (Fig. 3.6). Subcutaneous hemorrhage or petechiae, together with vascular engorgement, edema, and cyanosis of the head, neck, and upper extremities, are seen. This clinical picture is caused by an abrupt and sustained rise in pressure in the superior vena cava and hypoxemia attributable to hypoventilation caused by crushing of the chest. Although these patients often appear moribund initially, the neurological impairment resolves if the patient is rescued early. Sustained compression causes crushing death. There have been many reports of victims of crushing death and traumatic asphyxia in the setting of large earthquakes. Treatment of traumatic asphyxia is supportive.

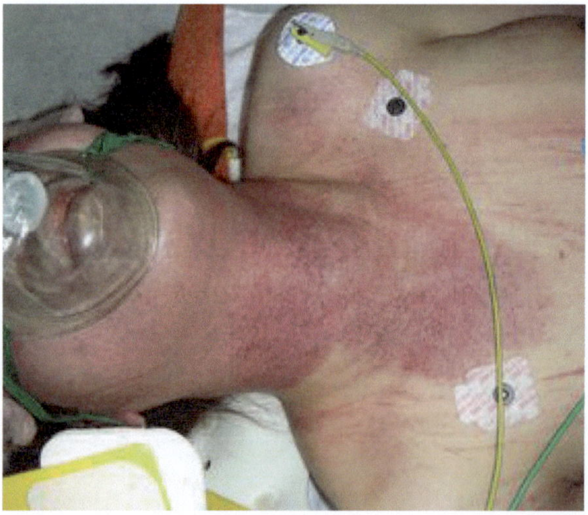

Fig. 3.6 Traumatic asphyxia in a woman who had become sandwiched inside a pressing machine. Just after she was rescued, she had dyspnea and was agitated and disoriented. Marked congestion of the face and neck and hemorrhage of conjunctiva were seen. She also had sternal and left humeral fractures. She was managed conservatively and discharged after 3 days with immediate recovery

3.7.2 *Crush Syndrome*

Crush syndrome is the second most common cause of death after direct trauma following major earthquakes. Up to 80% of crush victims die at the scene, 10% make an uneventful recovery, and the other 10% progress to crush syndrome [19]. Crush syndrome refers to systemic manifestations produced by extensive muscle damage in response to a direct physical crush injury (Fig. 3.7). Crush syndrome affects multiple organ systems, including the kidney and lung, and causes disseminated intravascular coagulation, hypovolemic shock, electrolyte abnormalities, and arrhythmias [20].

3.7.2.1 Pathophysiology

Reperfusion of damaged ischemic muscles starts when tension is released after the rescue. Crush syndrome is caused by the release of intracellular contents into the circulation, including myoglobin, lactic acid, uric acid, and muscle enzymes, such as creatine phosphokinase (CPK) and aldolase, in addition to ions, including like potassium, calcium, and phosphorus [3, 4].

Acute kidney injury (AKI) is the most serious complication of crush syndrome. Renal tubular obstruction occurs secondary to precipitation of myoglobin and uric acid. Crush-induced AKI may also occur as a result of hypovolemia, acidosis, and aciduria.

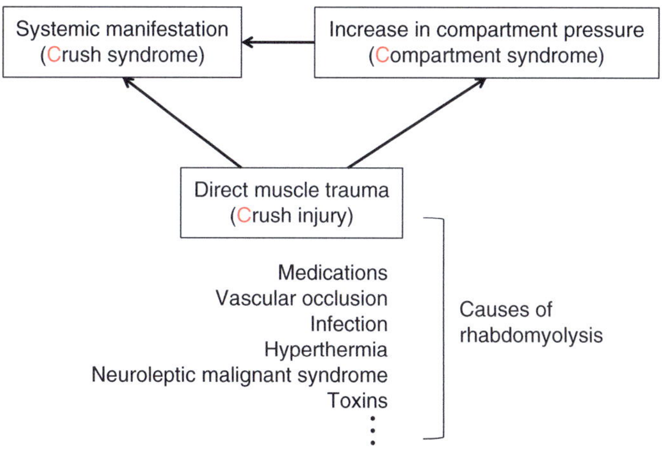

Fig. 3.7 Causal relationships among crush-related injuries

Multiple organ failure, including ARDS, often occurs in patients with crush syndrome. The mechanism of the effect of crush injury on distant organs has not been fully elucidated; however, systemic inflammation and endothelial damage may have some role [21].

Hyperkalemia, which occurs in response to release of potassium from injured skeletal muscle as well as renal dysfunction, can cause life-threatening cardiac arrhythmia. The serum phosphorus level may be elevated initially because of leakage of phosphorus from injured muscle tissue. Hypocalcemia often occurs as a result of deposition of calcium salts in necrotic muscle tissue. Later on, large calcifications are sometimes observed in the injured muscle. Disseminated intravascular coagulation frequently occurs and can result in hemorrhagic complications.

The affected muscle groups show marked swelling and edema. Inelastic fascial sheaths encase the skeletal muscles in the forearm and lower leg and are particularly vulnerable if there is a marked increase in compartment pressures, resulting in compartment syndrome. Massive swelling may not become apparent until after rehydration with intravenous fluids.

3.7.2.2 Clinical Features

Most crush victims are conscious at the time of rescue and deteriorate only after being rescued out of collapsed debris or from entrapment. Petechiae, blisters, muscle bruising, and superficial injuries are common. The affected muscles are grossly swollen, hard, cold, paralytic, and insensitive. Malaise, low-grade fever, and dark (tea- or cola-colored) urine are seen (Fig. 3.8). Nausea, vomiting, tachycardia, agitation, and delirium can be seen in severe cases. Soon afterward, these patients go into shock.

An elevated serum CPK is the traditional indicator of muscle injury. The degree of CPK elevation correlates with the amount of muscle injury and the severity of illness, but not with the development of AKI. The serum myoglobin level not only increases before the rise in serum CPK but also causes direct damage to the renal

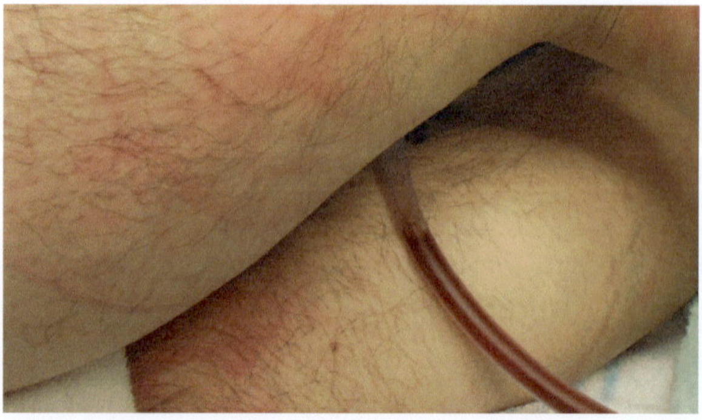

Fig. 3.8 Myoglobinuria in a patient with crush syndrome

tubules, leading to AKI. Therefore, it seems likely that serum myoglobin is the best diagnostic marker for crush syndrome.

3.7.2.3 Treatment

Resuscitation of crush victims should be started in the field. After adequate intravascular access is achieved, isotonic fluid replacement with normal saline should be started even before extrication of the crushed limb. If fluid therapy is delayed, the incidence of renal failure increases to 50%; delays of 12 h are associated with a 100% incidence.

On arrival in the emergency department, the mainstay of therapy is aggressive intravenous rehydration with isotonic saline. Potassium-containing solutions should be avoided. Intravenous fluid therapy can maximize the tubular flow rate, thereby avoiding accumulation of myoglobin in the renal tubules and aiding the clearance of hyperkalemia. Although fluid resuscitation is essential in the prevention of AKI, the treatment policy should be individualized [22]. Volume status and urine flow should be considered. Symptoms of fluid depletion, bleeding, and third spacing suggest hypovolemia, which necessitates administration of more fluids. Victims for whom the rescue is delayed often show no response to fluids and develop hypervolemia if excessive amounts of fluid are administered. Smaller volumes of fluid should be administered in patients with signs of hypervolemia, especially those with anuria. Excessive hypervolemia can cause pulmonary edema or aggravate ARDS, which frequently complicates crush syndrome.

Sodium bicarbonate has been recommended to maintain a urinary pH >6.5 for prevention of AKI. Some authorities recommend 50 mmol of bicarbonate per liter of isotonic saline. However, despite adequate treatment, dialysis may be indicated if aggressive fluid resuscitation fails. It should be emphasized that life-threatening complications are more frequent in patients with crush-related AKI than in those with AKI and other causes. Patients should be placed on a cardiac monitor because of the risk of dysrhythmia secondary to metabolic complications. Hyperkalemia, which is most severe in the first 12–36 h following a crush injury, can be fatal when associated with AKI. Treatment should be initiated to prevent cardiac complications. Traditional insulin and glucose therapy, although recommended, may not be as effective in crush-induced hyperkalemia because the potassium load is very high in such a situation. Ion-exchange resins (e.g., sodium polystyrene sulfonate) are effective, as is dialysis. Not only established hyperkalemia but also a rapidly increasing serum potassium level should be an indication for dialysis. There is a massive demand for dialysis machines in disaster settings.

Hypocalcemia observed early in crush syndrome should not be treated unless patients are symptomatic. Calcium should only be given to treat hyperkalemia-induced cardiotoxicity.

ARDS often occurs following crush syndrome. Treatment of ARDS is described in detail elsewhere [16].

3.8 Conclusion

Various kinds of respiratory system injuries occur in disaster settings and include traumatic thoracic injury, traumatic asphyxia, and inhalation injury. Further, multisystem injuries occur in combination with those sustained by the respiratory system. Poor hygiene, air and water pollution, malnutrition as a result of food shortage, and limited medical resources in a disaster setting can aggravate the course of disaster-related injuries. Huge numbers of casualties occur at the scene of a disaster. The principle in disaster medicine is to provide the best treatment to the greatest number of victims using limited medical resources [23]. Victims with severe injuries or complications who need a large amount of medical resources should be transported to facilities outside the disaster zone for further treatment after vital signs are stabilized.

To ensure an integrated and effective response to disasters in the future, physicians should understand the fundamental principles of disaster medicine and participate in the disaster planning process.

References

1. Ryan CM, Schoenfeld DA, Thorpe WP, Sheridan RL, Cassem EH, Tompkins RG. Objective estimates of the probability of death from burn injuries. N Engl J Med. 1998;338:362–6. https://doi.org/10.1056/NEJM199802053380604.
2. Toussaint J, Singer AJ. The evaluation and management of thermal injuries: 2014 update. Clin Exp Emerg Med. 2014;1:8–18. https://doi.org/10.15441/ceem.14.029.
3. Tintinalli JE, Stapczynski JS, Ma OJ, Cline DM, Cydulka RK, Meckler GD. Tintinalli's emergency medicine: a comprehensive study guide. 7th ed. New York: McGraw-Hill; 2011.
4. Vincent JL, Abraham E, Moore FA, Kochanek PM, Fink MP. Textbook of critical care. 6th ed. Philadelphia: Elsevier; 2011.
5. ISBI Practice Guidelines Committee; Steering Subcommittee; Advisory Subcommittee. ISBI practice guidelines for burn care. Burns. 2016;42:953–1021. https://doi.org/10.1016/j.burns.2016.05.013.
6. American Burn Association. Advanced burn life support course provider manual. Chicago: American Burn Association; 2011.
7. Mackie DP. Inhalation injury or mechanical ventilation: which is the true killer in burn patients? Burns. 2013;39:1329–30. https://doi.org/10.1016/j.burns.2013.07.006.
8. Monafo WW. Initial management of burns. N Engl J Med. 1996;335:1581–6. https://doi.org/10.1056/NEJM199611213352108.
9. Richardson JD. What's new in trauma and burns. J Am Coll Surg. 1997;184:210–6.
10. Galan G, Peñalver JC, París F, Caffarena JM Jr, Blasco E, Borro JM, et al. Blunt chest injuries in 1696 patients. Eur J Cardiothorac Surg. 1992;6:284–7.
11. American College of Surgeons Committee on Trauma. Advanced trauma life support for doctors: student course manual. 8th ed. Chicago: American College of Surgeons; 2008.
12. Morley EJ, Johnson S, Leibner E, Shahid J. Emergency department evaluation and management of blunt chest and lung trauma (Trauma CME). Emerg Med Pract. 2016;18:1–20.
13. Simon BJ, Cushman J, Barraco R, Lane V, Luchette FA, Miglietta M, et al. EAST Practice Management Guidelines Work Group. Pain management guidelines for blunt thoracic trauma. J Trauma. 2005;59:1256–67.

14. Barnea Y, Kashtan H, Skornick Y, Werbin N. Isolated rib fractures in elderly patients: mortality and morbidity. Can J Surg. 2002;45:43–6.
15. Cohn SM, Dubose JJ. Pulmonary contusion: an update on recent advances in clinical management. World J Surg. 2010;34:1959–70. https://doi.org/10.1007/s00268-010-0599-9.
16. Fan E, Del Sorbo L, Goligher EC, Hodgson CL, Munshi L, Walkey AJ, American Thoracic Society, European Society of Intensive Care Medicine, and Society of Critical Care Medicine, et al. An Official American Thoracic Society/European Society of Intensive Care Medicine/ Society of Critical Care Medicine Clinical Practice Guideline: Mechanical Ventilation in Adult Patients with Acute Respiratory Distress Syndrome. Am J Respir Crit Care Med. 2017;195:1253–63. https://doi.org/10.1164/rccm.201703-0548ST.
17. Simon B, Ebert J, Bokhari F, Capella J, Emhoff T, Hayward T 3rd, et al. Eastern Association for the Surgery of Trauma. Management of pulmonary contusion and flail chest: an Eastern Association for the Surgery of Trauma practice management guideline. J Trauma Acute Care Surg. 2012;73:S351–61. https://doi.org/10.1097/TA.0b013e31827019fd.
18. Jacobs JV, Hooft NM, Robinson BR, Todd E, Bremner RM, Petersen SR, et al. The use of extracorporeal membrane oxygenation in blunt thoracic trauma: a study of the Extracorporeal Life Support Organization database. J Trauma Acute Care Surg. 2015;79:1049–53.; discussion 1053–4. https://doi.org/10.1097/TA.0000000000000790.
19. Bywaters EG. 50 years on: the crush syndrome. BMJ. 1990;301:1412–5.
20. Sever MS, Vanholder R, Lameire N. Management of crush-related injuries after disasters. N Engl J Med. 2006;354:1052–63. https://doi.org/10.1056/NEJMra054329.
21. Sonoi H, Matsumoto N, Ogura H, Hosotsubo H, Noguchi K, Kuwagata Y, et al. The effect of antithrombin on pulmonary endothelial damage induced by crush injury. Shock. 2009;32:593–600. https://doi.org/10.1097/SHK.0b013e3181a23ad0.
22. Sever MS, Vanholder R. Management of crush victims in mass disasters: highlights from recently published recommendations. Clin J Am Soc Nephrol. 2013;8:328–35. https://doi.org/10.2215/CJN.07340712.
23. Russel R, Hodgetts TJ, Mahoney PF, Castle N. Disaster rules. Oxford: Blackwell; 2011.

Part II
Respiratory Disturbance by Aggravation of the Living Environment

Chapter 4
Respiratory Infection and Aggravation of Pulmonary Disease Related to Environmental Hygiene Aggravation: What Types of Respiratory Infection and Aggravation of Respiratory Diseases Are Increased by Aggravation of Environmental Hygiene?

Shinsuke Yamanda

Abstract After large-scale natural disasters, environmental hygiene in affected areas is aggravated by several causes. This aggravation of environmental hygiene leads to an increased incidence of respiratory infection and exacerbation of chronic pulmonary disease, such as acute respiratory infection, pneumonia, influenza, and tuberculosis; acute exacerbation of chronic obstructive pulmonary disease; and exacerbation of asthma.

Keywords Tsunami · Natural disaster · Respiratory infection · Respiratory disease Environmental hygiene

4.1 Introduction

Large-scale natural disasters, such as earthquakes and tsunamis, kill a significant number of people; this includes victims of direct chest trauma or aspiration of water [1, 2]. However, this is just one threat of natural disasters. Natural disasters also destroy individual residences as well as infrastructure (e.g., electricity, water, oil, communication, and transportation) and scatter dirty water and dust. This aggravates environmental hygiene, which is followed by an increase in respiratory infections and exacerbation of chronic respiratory disease [3]. This impact persists for months or years after the disasters.

S. Yamanda
Department of Respiratory Medicine, Sendai Kousei Hospital, Sendai, Japan

K. Fujimoto (ed.), *Disaster and Respiratory Diseases*,
Respiratory Disease Series: Diagnostic Tools and Disease Managements,
https://doi.org/10.1007/978-981-13-2598-4_4

This aggravation of environmental hygiene after the disasters occurs in both industrial countries and developed countries. The consequences of devastating disasters such as Hurricane Katrina in the USA (2005) and the Great East Japan Earthquake (2011) have shown that even the most developed countries are vulnerable to natural disasters [4, 5]. These disasters help provide information to help develop countermeasures to mitigate the effects of future disasters. In this chapter, the impact of aggravation of environmental hygiene after the natural disasters on respiratory disease is discussed.

4.2 Aggravation of Respiratory Diseases due to Deterioration of Environmental Hygiene After Natural Disasters

The following classification scheme, consisting of three clinical phases of natural disasters, has been proposed to guide adequate relief efforts and countermeasures to reduce the effects of disasters (Table 4.1) [6]. Although this classification scheme was initially used in the field of infectious disease, it is also useful to guide understanding regarding the impact of natural disasters on environmental hygiene and respiratory disease.

The impact phase (lasting 0–4 days) is usually the period when victims are extricated and provided initial treatment for disaster-related injuries and diseases. The postimpact phase (4 days to 4 weeks) is the period when the first waves of infectious disease (airborne, foodborne, and waterborne infections) emerge. The recovery phase (after 4 weeks) is the period when symptoms may become clinically apparent in victims who have contracted infections with long incubation periods or those with latent-type infections. However, it must be emphasized that this timeline is not absolute and represents some degree of overlap, especially phase 2 and phase 3. The more devastating the disaster, the longer the phases 2 and 3 are. Moreover, they differ by specific situations, such as developed or developing country and warm or cold area.

4.2.1 *The Impact Phase (0–4 Days)*

Natural disasters destroy a variety of types of infrastructure, followed by collapse of health facilities and healthcare systems, as well as by disruption of surveillance and health programs. Earthquake-caused building collapses and fires cause air pollution, whereas invasion of water by tsunami or flood brings contaminants into residential areas. However, these events do not affect victims in this period.

Table 4.1 Classification of periods after natural disasters

	Classification	Timeline
Phase 1	Impact phase	0–4 days
Phase 2	Postimpact phase	4 days to 4 weeks
Phase 3	Recovery phase	After 4 weeks

4.2.2 The Postimpact Phase (4 Days to 4 Weeks)

In this period, a great number of survivors are displaced from their residences to overcrowded shelters. These shelters usually have poor ventilation systems and a shortage of water and sanitary goods, resulting in poor personal hygiene. Acute respiratory infection due to viral infection, pneumonia, asthma, acute exacerbation of chronic obstructive pulmonary disease (COPD), and other communicable respiratory diseases emerge in this phase [4, 7–9].

4.2.3 The Recovery Phase (After 4 Weeks)

Some refugees return and restart their lives in their residences, which have been partially destroyed and contaminated with sediments deposited by tsunami or flood waters and subsequently by microbial overgrowth, especially fungi; others move to temporary housing or stay in shelters where indoor mold counts typically increase. Individuals engaging in restoration work are at risk of inhalation exposure to dust containing microbial and other agents. Exacerbation and new onsets of asthma, allergic bronchopulmonary aspergillosis, hypersensitivity pneumonitis, toxic alveolitis, and pneumonia are elicited in these situations [5, 10, 11].

4.3 Respiratory Diseases and Aggravation of Environmental Hygiene After Natural Disaster

4.3.1 Acute Respiratory Infection

Epidemics of acute respiratory infection (ARI), the most common communicable disease that sometimes includes pneumonia, have often been reported after natural disasters. ARI often occurs in the first 3–5 days following the disaster and is associated with inadequate protection during cold winter nights. To prevent outbreak of ARI, adequate space of 4.5–5.5 m^2/person in shelters is recommended [1, 2, 12].

4.3.2 Pneumonia in the Elderly

A significant increase in pneumonia hospitalization and death has been reported from Japan. After the Hanshin-Awaji Earthquake (1995) and Great East Japan Earthquake, numerous individuals, primarily elderly people with physical and mental limitations, were hospitalized for pneumonia. The causative pathogens of pneumonia leading to hospitalization after the disaster were similar to those before the disaster: *Streptococcus pneumoniae* was the most common pathogen, followed by *Haemophilus influenzae*, *Moraxella catarrhalis*, and *Klebsiella pneumoniae*.

A lack of appropriate nutrition, absence of caregivers, and shortage of water lead to deterioration of activities of daily living and poor oral hygiene in elderly individuals. Poor activities of daily living and loss of oral hygiene are major risk factors for pneumonia. As sufficient supplies of water and other sanitary goods cannot be expected in many cases, elderly individuals should be moved to other places, such as temporary housing or nursing homes in non-affected areas [4, 13–15].

4.3.3 Influenza

Influenza outbreaks can take place in post-disaster settings when disasters occur during an epidemic season. Overcrowding of shelters, inadequate ventilation, and poor hand hygiene due to the disrupted water supply are risk factors for outbreaks. Patient isolation, active case finding, strong promotion of hand hygiene and mask-wearing, and postexposure prophylaxis should be implemented in these settings [16, 17].

4.3.4 Tuberculosis

Refugees and populations displaced after natural disasters are vulnerable to tuberculosis because crowded living conditions and poor nutritional status can facilitate its development and transmission. Moreover, poor access to medical institutions in affected areas delays access to medical care. Improving educational efforts in relation to health concerns regarding tuberculosis is necessary in affected areas [18, 19].

4.3.5 Asthma

Natural disasters, especially tsunamis and floods, increase the mold concentration in the surrounding environment. Exposure to this and other contaminants can exacerbate existing asthma, and there is mounting evidence that such exposures increase the risk of developing new asthma. Individuals should be protected against these microbial exposures by using dust control measures and appropriate personal protective equipment [4, 5, 10, 11].

4.3.6 Acute Exacerbation of COPD

An increase in an acute exacerbation of COPD after earthquakes has primarily been reported from Japan. Respiratory infections and air pollution are important risk factors for an acute exacerbation of COPD. In addition, because patients with COPD are generally older, they are more vulnerable in the post-disaster setting [20].

4.4 Conclusion

After natural disasters, an aggravation of environmental hygiene causes an increase in the incidence of infectious and noninfectious respiratory diseases. These diseases are not particular to the post-disaster setting but are suppressed by the power of public hygiene before the disasters.

References

1. Robinson B, Alatas MF, Robertson A, Steer H. Natural disasters and the lung. Respirology. 2011;16(3):386–95.
2. Kouadio IK, Aljunid S, Kamigaki T, Hammad K, Oshitani H. Infectious diseases following natural disasters: prevention and control measures. Expert Rev Anti-Infect Ther. 2012;10(1):95–104.
3. Sato H, Tomio J. Emergency and disaster preparedness for chronically ill patients: a review of recommendations. Open Access Emerg Med. 2014;6:69.
4. Yamanda S, Hanagama M, Kobayashi S, Satou H, Tokuda S, Niu K, Yanai M. The impact of the 2011 Great East Japan Earthquake on hospitalisation for respiratory disease in a rapidly aging society: a retrospective descriptive and cross-sectional study at the disaster base hospital in Ishinomaki. BMJ Open. 2013;3(1):e000865.
5. Rando RJ, Lefante JJ, Freyder LM, Jones RN. Respiratory health effects associated with restoration work in post-hurricane katrina New Orleans. J Environ Public Health. 2012;2012:462478.
6. Aghababian RV, Teuscher J. Infectious diseases following major disasters. Ann Emerg Med. 1992;21(4):362–7.
7. Nukiwa T. An overview of respiratory medicine during the Tsunami Disaster at Tohoku, Japan, on March 11, 2011. Respir Investig. 2012;50(4):124–8.
8. Ohkouchi S, Shibuya R, Yanai M, Kikuchi Y, Ichinose M, Nukiwa T. Deterioration in regional health status after the acute phase of a great disaster: respiratory physicians' experiences of the Great East Japan Earthquake. Respir Investig. 2013;51(2):50–5.
9. Takakura R, Himeno S, Kanayama Y, Sonoda T, Kiriyama K, Furubayashi T, Yabu M, Yoshida S, Nagasawa Y, Inoue S, Iwao N. Follow-up after the Hanshin-Awaji earthquake: diverse influences on pneumonia, bronchial asthma, peptic ulcer and diabetes mellitus. Intern Med. 1997;36(2):87–91.
10. Oshikata C, Watanabe M, Saito A, Ishida M, Kobayashi S, Konuma R, Kamata Y, Terajima J, Cho J, Yanai M, Tsurikisawa N. Allergic bronchopulmonary mycosis due to exposure to Eurotium herbariorum after the Great East Japan Earthquake. Prehosp Disaster Med. 2017;32(6):688–90.
11. Johanning E, Auger P, Morey PR, Yang CS, Olmsted E. Review of health hazards and prevention measures for response and recovery workers and volunteers after natural disasters, flooding, and water damage: Mold and dampness. Environ Health Prev Med. 2014;19(2):93–9.
12. Kawano T, Tsugawa Y, Nishiyama K, Morita H, Yamamura O, Hasegawa K. Shelter crowding and increased incidence of acute respiratory infection in evacuees following the Great Eastern Japan Earthquake and tsunami. Epidemiol Infect. 2016;144(4):787–95.
13. Aoyagi T, Yamada M, Kunishima H, Tokuda K, Yano H, Ishibashi N, Hatta M, Endo S, Arai K, Inomata S, Gu Y, Kanamori H, Kitagawa M, Hirakata Y, Kaku M. Characteristics of infectious diseases in hospitalized patients during the early phase after the 2011 Great East Japan Earthquake. Chest. 2013;143(2):349–56.
14. Daito H, Suzuki M, Shiihara J, Kilgore PE, Ohtomo H, Morimoto K, Ishida M, Kamigaki T, Oshitani H, Hashizume M, Endo W, Hagiwara K, Ariyoshi K, Okinaga S. Impact of the Tohoku earthquake and tsunami on pneumonia hospitalisations and mortality among adults in northern Miyagi, Japan: a multicentre observational study. Thorax. 2013;68(6):544–50.

15. Shibata Y, Ojima T, Tomata Y, Okada E, Nakamura M, Kawado M, Hashimoto S. Characteristics of pneumonia deaths after an earthquake and tsunami: an ecological study of 5.7 million participants in 131 municipalities, Japan. BMJ Open. 2016;6(2):1–6.
16. Kamigaki T, Seino J, Tohma K, Nukiwa-Soma N, Otani K, Oshitani H. Investigation of an Influenza A (H3N2) outbreak in evacuation centres following the Great East Japan earthquake, 2011. BMC Public Health. 2014;14(1):34.
17. Hatta M, Endo S, Tokuda K, Kunishima H, Arai K, Yano H, Ishibashi N, Aoyagi T, Yamada M, Inomata S, Kanamori H, Gu Y, Kitagawa M, Hirakata Y, Kaku M. Post-tsunami outbreaks of influenza in evacuation centers in Miyagi Prefecture, Japan. Clin Infect Dis. 2012;54(1):e5–7.
18. Kanamori H, Hatakeyama T, Uchiyama B, Weber DJ, Takeuchi M, Endo S, Hirakata Y, Kaku M. Clinical and molecular epidemiological features of tuberculosis after the 2011 Japan earthquake and tsunami. Int J Tuberc Lung Dis. 2016;20(4):505–14.
19. Kanamori H, Aso N, Tadano S, Saito M, Saito H, Uchiyama B, Ishibashi N, Inomata S, Endo S, Aoyagi T, Hatta M, Yamada M, Gu Y, Tokuda K, Yano H, Kunishima H, Hirakata Y, Saijyo T, Kitagawa M, Kaku M. Tuberculosis exposure among evacuees at a shelter after earthquake, Japan, 2011. Emerg Infect Dis. 2013;19(5):799–801.
20. Kobayashi S, Hanagama M, Yamanda S, Satoh H, Tokuda S, Kobayashi M, Ueda S, Suzuki S, Yanai M. The impact of a large-scale natural disaster on patients with chronic obstructive pulmonary disease: the aftermath of the 2011 Great East Japan Earthquake. Respir Investig. 2013;51(1):17–23.

Chapter 5
Aggravation of Asthma by Cold, Fatigue, Stress, or Discontinuation of Medicines: What Should We Measures and Prevents Worse of Asthma Control Induced by the Aggravation of the Environmental Hygiene and/or the Stopping Medicine?

Toshiyuki Koya and Takashi Hasegawa

Abstract Bronchial asthma can be exacerbated by many factors, the most important of which are airway infection, including upper respiratory tract infection. However, in times of disaster, changes in temperature (cold air), fatigue, mental stress, and discontinuation of medicines can also exacerbate asthma and cause acute symptoms. In such situations, clinicians often encounter the exacerbation of asthma symptoms by cold air, which is thought to affect the immune and nervous systems through contact with the airway mucosa. Deterioration of asthma due to fatigue and mental stress is also common. In particular, evacuation after disasters causes great mental stress, as do loss of home, uncertainty about the unpredictable future, etc. Medical system collapse and subsequent discontinuation of drug treatment are serious problems for patients with chronic disease. In particular, inhaled corticosteroids are critical medicines for asthma patients. Maintaining a system of drug supply after major disasters is a challenge in Japan, which experiences many natural disasters, including earthquakes.

Keywords Cold air · Physical fatigue · Mental stress · Inhaled corticosteroid · Asthma death

---

T. Koya (✉)
Department of Respiratory Medicine and Infectious Diseases, Niigata University Graduate School of Medical and Dental Sciences, Niigata City, Niigata, Japan
e-mail: tkoya@med.niigata-u.ac.jp

T. Hasegawa
Department of General Medicine, Niigata University Medical and Dental Hospital, Niigata City, Niigata, Japan

K. Fujimoto (ed.), *Disaster and Respiratory Diseases*,
Respiratory Disease Series: Diagnostic Tools and Disease Managements,
https://doi.org/10.1007/978-981-13-2598-4_5

5.1 Introduction

Exacerbation of bronchial asthma at times of disaster is an important topic. Several studies have reported that patients' asthma control deteriorated after major earthquakes and disasters [1–3], although another publication stated that asthma was unaffected in such situations [4]. In this chapter, we explain how asthma can be exacerbated by changes in temperature (cold air: chillness), fatigue, stress, and discontinuation of medication, all of which can be encountered after a disaster.

5.2 Chillness

After natural disasters, residents are often forced to evacuate to ensure their survival. In general, evacuation facilities are insufficiently equipped and poorly stocked with necessary products such as food and medicines. Furthermore, temperature and humidity are often poorly controlled, as is hygiene. Sudden temperature changes are likely, especially when the weather worsens. Moreover, to avoid living in shelters, many people, especially the younger generation, live in their cars, which are difficult environment to adjust temperature change.

Weather changes have long been known to exacerbate asthma, and the disease often deteriorates after a typhoon or cold front [5]. Of particular importance is the effect of cold air, which tends to worsen symptoms in cases of poor asthma control [6] and cough-variant asthma [7]. One Hong Kong study showed an inverse correlation between temperature and asthma hospitalization during winter, with low humidity leading to further hospitalization [8]. In a Taiwan study conducted over 10 years from 2000 to 2009, Wang et al. analyzed the relationship between the risk of emergency room visit and temperature in patients with chronic disease [9]. They reported that, in bronchial asthma and obstructive pulmonary disease, higher temperatures were associated with a lower risk of emergency outpatient visits, while lower temperatures conferred a higher risk. In another study involving childhood asthma, rapid changes in weather were reported to be important. Hashimoto et al. analyzed the relationship between emergency room visits and weather over 5 years. They reported that decreases in atmospheric pressure, temperature, and humidity were related to the risk of emergency room visits by asthmatic children within 3 days, especially in spring and autumn [10].

Cold air can exacerbate asthma symptoms via several mechanisms, including direct contact between cold air and the respiratory tract, which causes the temperature of the airway mucosa to drop, leading to dryness, changes in the osmotic pressure of airway mucus, activation of the nervous system, release of inflammatory mediators from mast cells, and airway contraction [11, 12]. Neutrophils may also be involved. The immune system weakens in cold temperatures. However, corticosteroid secretion increases, as does the accumulation of neutrophils in the respiratory tract. Inflammatory mediators released by neutrophils injure the airway epithelium and cause airway contraction, which can lead to asthma exacerbation [13]. Older patients are reported to be particularly sensitive to cold air [8].

To prevent asthma exacerbation by cold air, it is important to prevent exposure by maintaining room temperature. Masks are another effective way of preventing direct intrusion of cold air; they are also effective for exercise-induced asthma, which is also exacerbated by cold air [14].

5.3 Fatigue

Evacuees of natural disasters are prone to physical and mental fatigue. In this section, we will explain physical fatigue, while the next section will focus on the mental fatigue caused by stress. After natural disasters, victims must engage in various difficult manual tasks. For example, they must demolish collapsed houses, tidy up home furnishings, purchase supplies, etc. In addition, fear of aftershocks, and insomnia caused by unfamiliar sleeping environments, can spur exhaustion. In fact, one previous report [15] stated that asthma was exacerbated by overwork after an earthquake.

Few reports have described the effects of fatigue on asthma. However, in clinical practice, fatigue and overwork are often cited as causes of exacerbation. One questionnaire survey of asthma death conducted among physicians in Japan found that fatigue and overwork affect asthma, as do respiratory tract infections and stress [16, 17]. Thus, it is important that patients rest properly during asthma management.

The mechanisms of asthma exacerbation due to fatigue are unclear. Several factors are thought to overlap, including physiological mechanisms, increases in mental stress, decreases in adherence to therapeutic agents, and underestimation of symptoms.

5.4 Stress

Evacuation after a natural disaster causes great mental stress [18, 19]. Moreover, in disasters that cause many deaths, guilt and grief often progress to depression in survivors [20].

In around 400 BC, Hippocrates pointed out that psychological factors are involved in asthma. More recently, it was reported that psychosocial stress causes asthma onset, exacerbation, poor treatment management, etc.—both in children [21] and adults [22]. One experimental study reported that viewing of short films induced various emotions such as anxiety, anger, depression, elation, and happiness and induced significant increases in airway resistance in asthma patients. These data indicate that changes in emotion and stress are associated with airway contraction [23, 24]. Another study evaluated airway inflammation using the allergen provocation test in university students with mild asthma during a week with a test and a week without. The data showed a significant increase in the number of inflammatory cells, particularly eosinophils, in the sputum during the week with the test; furthermore, the eosinophil fraction in the sputum correlated with the change in respiratory function [25]. One psychiatric evaluation (Patient Health Questionnaire-9: PHQ-9) reported that 3.4% of suspected major depressive disorders and 2.4% of suspected other depressive disorders were present in patients with asthma [26].

With regard to the relationship between depression and asthma control, patients with depression often overestimate their symptoms. Previously, we conducted an asthma control test (ACT) and PHQ-9 on asthma patients. We compared ACT scores between patients with depression and those without, thereby creating a true control situation, as defined by the Global Initiative for Asthma (GINA) [27]. The study found that the threshold ACT score indicating good control was 23 in patients without depression but lower than 20 in patients with depression, indicating that patients with depression tend to overreport symptoms (Fig. 5.1a, b). Nonetheless, there are many cases of poor control in patients with depression, so clinicians risk mischaracterizing their patient's condition as an overestimation of symptoms.

Mental stress is associated with the hypothalamic-pituitary-adrenocortical axis and sympathetic-adrenomedullary system, which secrete the stress hormones cortisol and catecholamine, respectively. These stress hormones shift the immune response from a Th1 type to a Th2 type by suppressing production of Th1 cytokines like IL-12. Stress also promotes production of endogenous opioids; subsequent activation of μ-opioid receptors induces Th2 cell differentiation and promotes a shift from the Th1-type to the Th2-type immune response [28]. Stress-related neuropeptides may also play a role in regulating airway inflammation.

Regarding the influence of asthma on mental stress after a disaster, many reports have focused on the terrorist attacks on the World Trade Center (WTC) on September

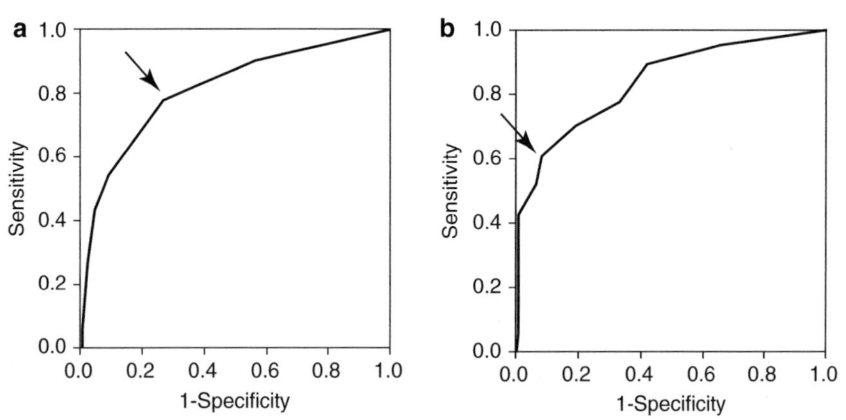

Fig. 5.1 Receiver operating characteristic curve of the ACT score for assessing uncontrolled asthma in the non-depressive group (**a**) and the depressive group (**b**). The area under the curve was 0.821 (95% confidence interval (CI), 0.801–0.843) in the non-depressive group and 0.846 (95% CI, 0.807–0.885) in the depressive group. The optimal cutoff points were 23 in the non-depressive group and 20 in the depressive group

11, 2001. In a phone survey conducted 5–9 weeks later, 27% of patients with asthma claimed they had experienced stronger symptoms after the attack. The same report warned that breathing problems can be caused by smoke and debris, as well as by intense mental distress [29].

In a study of adults who had experienced the attack on the WTC, Brackbill et al. investigated the association between the post-traumatic stress (PTS) and bronchial asthma. The investigation reported that 10.2% of respondents had newly developed asthma and that there was a high asthma incidence among rescue workers and restoration workers in nearby offices. Patients experiencing PTS symptoms also had high asthma incidence rates [30]. Furthermore, an observational study conducted among rescue and restoration workers 9 years after the incident revealed a 27.6% incidence of asthma, as well as a high incidence of psychological disorders such as depression and panic disorder [31].

With regard to long-term observations, 181 men with asthma who had worked in rescue and restoration at the WTC were examined for mental stress between December 2013 and April 2015. The study found that 28% of the patients had post-traumatic stress (PTSD) and that 25% of them were close to PTSD. Patients with PTSD had poorer asthma control that those without. As a result, they often required hospitalization and had a decreased quality of life [32]. Thus, even though it had been more than 10 years since the incident, patients continued to have serious mental stress that affected their asthma control.

Few reports have investigated the effects of mental stress and asthma after an earthquake. However, one survey was carried out in the Fukushima Prefecture after the Great East Japan Earthquake. In this prefecture, the accident at the Fukushima Daiichi Nuclear Power Plant overlapped with the earthquake. Mental stress was increased because people carried concerns about repeated aftershocks and damage to their houses. They were also worried because their daily lives had been interrupted by the earthquake, and they feared radiation contamination from the nuclear power plant. One study used the visual analog scale (VAS) to survey anxiety about the disaster and relate it to asthma status. The study showed that the VAS score for anxiety about asthma symptoms, asthma control, and asthma deterioration significantly increased in the group that felt anxiety about the disaster [33].

5.5 Discontinuation of Medicines

Medicines may be discontinued after natural disasters for various reasons. For example, the supply of anti-asthma medicine to patients can cease due to medical system collapse. Interruption of treatment due to the cessation of drug supply is a critical problem in most chronic diseases and is particularly important in hypertension, diabetes, and diseases requiring anticoagulant therapy. In addition, adherence to medication decreases due to mental stress in evacuation shelters, where victims are forced into collective living and are grieving the loss of friends and family members. Patients with bronchial asthma must continue using inhaled corticosteroids (ICSs), but this can become difficult when natural disasters occur.

Poor adherence, interruption, and inappropriate use of therapeutic drugs are widely known as risk factors for asthma exacerbation. In particular, the rate of asthma exacerbation is directly correlated with a decrease in adherence to ICSs and ICS/long-acting inhaled β2 agonist (LABA) combined therapy [34, 35]. Jentzsch et al. started ICS treatment in patients with asthma who had no history of steroid therapy, continuing the prescription for 1 year. Adherence to the ICSs was periodically measured electronically. The control status of asthma was defined using the GINA standards. In patients with good control, ICS adherence was 60.8% after 4 months but decreased to 49.8% after 12 months. Meanwhile, ICS adherence in patients with poor control was 43.8% after 4 months and 31.2% after 12 months. Furthermore, in multivariate analysis, ICS adherence was independently correlated with asthma control; thus, the research indicated that ICS adherence directly affected asthma control [34]. In a retrospective study using a database, Marceau et al. analyzed the association between adherence and therapeutic effect in patients using either an ICS/LABA combination or ICS and LABA concurrent use. Adherence was calculated based on the prescribed drug dose, and the therapeutic effect was evaluated by analyzing decreases in more than moderate exacerbation. Adherence to the ICS/LABA combination was better than to ICS and LABA concurrent use, and the therapeutic effect was significantly higher with the ICS/LABA combination than with ICS and LABA concurrent use [35].

It is difficult to analyze discontinuation of ICS in patients with childhood bronchial asthma. Zheug et al. observed patients whose clinical symptoms had been controlled for 3 years. They divided the patients into two groups: ICS discontinued and ICS continued. They then observed before and after follow-up, sputum eosinophil count, total IgE level, respiratory function, and airway hyper-responsiveness (provocation causing a 20% fall in FEV_1: PC_{20}) [36]. They found that PC_{20} was significantly lower in both groups but that the groups did not differ significantly in this regard. Sputum eosinophil count and serum IgE values were significantly higher in the in ICS discontinued group than in the ICS continued group, even though symptom control was good. These data suggest that airway hyper-responsiveness and inflammation cannot be controlled by ICS discontinuation.

Accurate execution of inhaler techniques is essential in inhalation therapy. However, in the elderly, mastering of the techniques is not easy. In particular, Japan is aging rapidly at unprecedented speed in other countries, and it is an urgent task to enrich medical care for the elderly. It is important to periodically repeat inhalation instruction for the elderly, which also leads to better medication adherence. However, such inhalation instruction cannot be performed only by medical institutions; it is necessary to cooperate with dispensing pharmacies and visiting nursing and elderly nursing care facilities. It is important to build the systems for inhalation instruction among facilities surrounding the elderly are in comprehensive medical care.

With regard to asthma death, a questionnaire survey delivered to physicians in Japan found that discontinuation of medicine is important, accounting for an 8% in asthma death [17].

After the Great East Japan Earthquake, patients who discontinued ICS use had increased asthma exacerbation, suggesting that it is important to re-establish drug supply systems after a large disaster [33]. Thus, the Japanese government allowed pharmacists to prescribe regular medicine without prescription if the patient regularly used the medicine. This emergency political measure was successful, and most patients with chronic disease had no interruption in the supply of drugs. Suzuki et al. relayed the state of asthma examinations after the Chuetsu Earthquake of 2004 [4]. Although the earthquake caused major damage, most patients still received their necessary medicines, and most were using ICS properly. Patients were also educated. In the 3 months after the earthquake, the number of asthma exacerbations had not increased more than in the normal year.

These data suggest that discontinuation or lower adherence to medication, including ICSs, is important in asthma control, especially in disaster situations. As a step to the elderly society, incorporating inhalation instruction and confirmation of medication into the regional comprehensive medical system are extremely important in considering future medical care for the elderly.

5.6 Questionnaire Survey on Exacerbation of Asthma

Chillness, fatigue, stress, and discontinuation of medicines, as described so far, are important causes of asthma exacerbation. Although respiratory tract infection is generally considered to be the most important cause of exacerbation, we previously conducted a questionnaire survey on asthma patients and recorded which factors they themselves consider to be important [37].

One study gave questionnaires to 3085 patients who visited the medical institutes of the Niigata Prefecture monthly from September through October 2006. The study stratified the patients by sex, age, disease type, and disease severity and analyzed factors contributing to asthma exacerbation, as described in the guideline of the Japanese Society of Allergology [38]. The following factors were found to be significant contributors: air pollutants, respiratory infection, exercise, smoking, weather, food and food additives, drugs, emotional stress, stimulants, sulfur dioxide, menstruation, pregnancy, obesity, alcohol, and fatigue. The study subjects were mostly, though not overwhelmingly, women (55.0%). The patients' mean age was 57.5 years. Among the subjects, 423 (13.8%) were current smokers.

The most important factor associated with asthma exacerbation, according to the patients, was weather. Emotional stress and fatigue were also major factors. Although respiratory infection is one of the most prevalent factors resulting in asthma exacerbation, it was ranked seventh in the questionnaire study. Respiratory infection, weather, and emotional stress were especially common exacerbating factors in women (Fig. 5.2). Furthermore, emotional stress was a more prominent factor in younger participants, whereas fatigue was a prominent factor in middle-aged subjects. With regard to disease severity, "allergen exposure," "drugs," "stimulants," and "obesity" were conspicuously present in patients with severe asthma, whereas "weather" and "emotional stress" were significantly less common in patients with mild disease (Fig. 5.3).

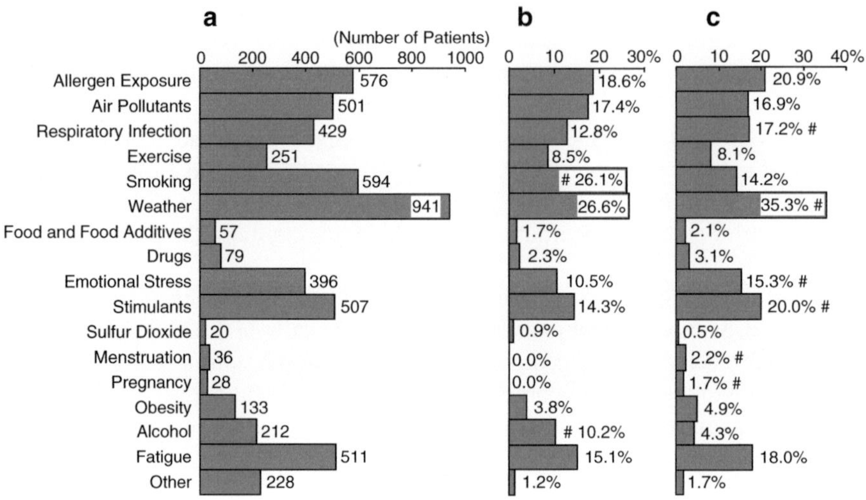

Fig. 5.2 Factors that exacerbated asthma in all applicants ($n = 3085$) (**a**) and percentages of factors that exacerbated asthma in male ($n = 1308$) (**b**) and female patients ($n = 1686$) (**c**). (**a**) Data are shown as the sum of multiple answers. (**b** and **c**) $^{\#}P < 0.01$ between the male and female groups

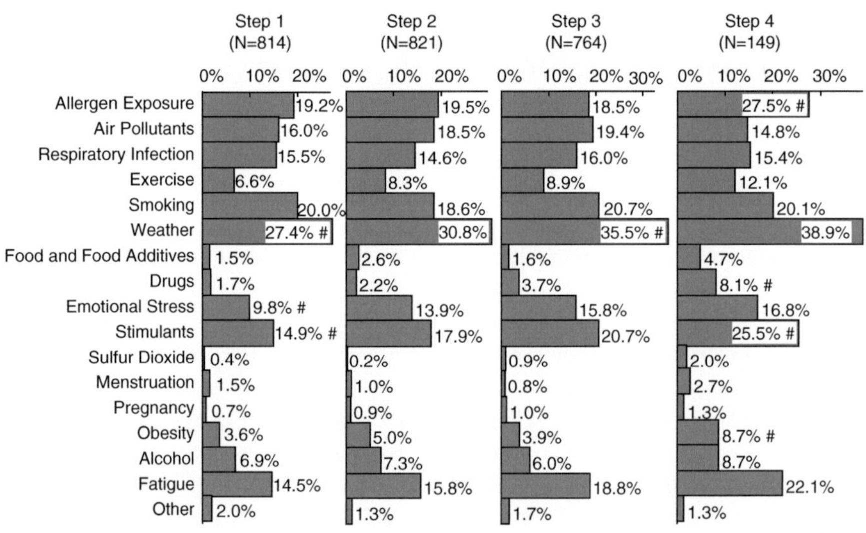

Fig. 5.3 Percentages of factors that exacerbated asthma, as defined using the Japanese Society of Allergology guideline. $^{\#}P < 0.01$ among the remaining groups

Table 5.1 Multiple regression analysis comparing weather changes to 11 independent factors

	RC	SE	SRC	*t*-value	*P*-value
Intercept	0.231	0.055	0.231	4.239	<0.0001
Duration	0.075	0.029	0.076	2.57	0.0103
Severity	0.008	0.015	0.016	0.562	0.5741
Disease type	0.013	0.028	0.012	0.453	0.651
Asthma in childhood	0.042	0.033	0.037	1.256	0.2092
Smoking	−0.055	0.018	−0.083	−3.104	0.002
OCS use	0.029	0.05	0.017	0.588	0.5568
PA (1 year)	0.097	0.022	0.143	4.351	<0.0001
PA (2 weeks)	0.072	0.037	0.066	1.948	0.0516
Admission	0.09	0.028	0.01	0.338	0.7356
AIA	0.01	0.049	0.005	0.196	0.8448
Satisfaction with daily life	0.006	0.019	0.009	0.324	0.7459

OCS oral corticosteroid, *PA (1 year)* patients experiencing asthma attacks during the year prior to answering the questionnaire, *PA (2 weeks)* patients experiencing asthma attacks during the 2 weeks prior to answering the questionnaire, *AIA* aspirin intolerant asthma, *RC* regression coefficient, *SE* standard error, *SRC* standardized regression coefficient

To determine other factors that were associated with weather, a multiple regression analysis was performed, which found that disease duration, poor asthma control during the last year, and current smoking were associated with weather (Table 5.1).

These data indicate that cold, fatigue, and stress are important in asthma exacerbation, even as reported by the patient. Furthermore, the importance of these factors seems to increase during disasters.

5.7 Conclusion

Various factors are known to exacerbate bronchial asthma. However, chillness (weather changes), fatigue, stress, and discontinuation of medicine are important in practical clinics. Furthermore, in the state of confusion that surrounds a disaster, the importance of these factors increases, and continuation of drugs is considered the most important among them in such situations. After the Great East Japan Earthquake, a lot of lives were lost, and many people were forced to evacuate—not only because of earthquake itself but also because of radiation pollution caused by the tsunami and the nuclear power plant accident. Many asthma patients who lived in evacuation accommodation for a long time felt that the shelters were a harsh environment and that the environmental changes caused physical fatigue and mental distress. However, several reports have stated that interruption of medication was not a big problem, because the government responded promptly and pharmaceutical companies offered aid as distribution routes became a problem. Because Japan suffers disasters often, its clinicians must prepare countermeasures that differ from routine clinical practice.

References

1. Tomita K, Hasegawa Y, Watanabe M, Sano H, Hitsuda Y, Shimizu E. The Totton-Ken Seibu earthquake and exacerbation of asthma in adults. J Med Investig. 2005;52(1–2):80–4.
2. Ishiura Y, Fujimura M, Yamamoto H, Shiba Y, Ohkura N, Kasahara K, et al. Asthma exacerbations after the East Japan Disaster. J Med Investig. 2013;60(1–2):61–5.
3. Yamanda S, Hanagama M, Kobayashi S, Satou H, Tokuda S, Niu K, et al. The impact of the 2011 Great East Japan Earthquake on hospitalisation for respiratory disease in a rapidly aging society: a retrospective descriptive and cross-sectional study at the disaster base hospital in Ishinomaki. BMJ Open. 2013;3(1) https://doi.org/10.1136/bmjopen-2012-000865.
4. Suzuki K, Hasegawa T, Iguchi S, Ota K, Sakagami T, Gejyo F, et al. The impact of the Chuetsu earthquake on asthma control. Allergol Int. 2007;56(2):179. https://doi.org/10.2332/allergolint.L-06-07.
5. Sato S, Saito J, Suzuki Y, Uematsu M, Fukuhara A, Togawa R, et al. Association between typhoon and asthma symptoms in Japan. Respir Investig. 2016;54(3):216–9. https://doi.org/10.1016/j.resinv.2015.10.002.
6. Hyrkas H, Ikaheimo TM, Jaakkola JJ, Jaakkola MS. Asthma control and cold weather-related respiratory symptoms. Respir Med. 2016;113:1–7. https://doi.org/10.1016/j.rmed.2016.02.005.
7. Kanemitsu Y, Matsumoto H, Osman N, Oguma T, Nagasaki T, Izuhara Y, et al. "Cold air" and/or "talking" as cough triggers, a sign for the diagnosis of cough variant asthma. Respir Investig. 2016;54(6):413–8. https://doi.org/10.1016/j.resinv.2016.07.002.
8. Lam HC, Li AM, Chan EY, Goggins WB 3rd. The short-term association between asthma hospitalisations, ambient temperature, other meteorological factors and air pollutants in Hong Kong: a time-series study. Thorax. 2016;71(12):1097–109. https://doi.org/10.1136/thoraxjnl-2015-208054.
9. Wang YC, Lin YK. Association between temperature and emergency room visits for cardiorespiratory diseases, metabolic syndrome-related diseases, and accidents in metropolitan Taipei. PLoS One. 2014;9(6):e99599. https://doi.org/10.1371/journal.pone.0099599.
10. Hashimoto M, Fukuda T, Shimizu T, Watanabe S, Watanuki S, Eto Y, et al. Influence of climate factors on emergency visits for childhood asthma attack. Pediatr Int. 2004;46(1):48–52. https://doi.org/10.1111/j.1442-200X.2004.01835.x.
11. Mustafa SM, Pilcher CW, Williams KI. Cooling-induced contraction in ovine airways smooth muscle. Pharmacol Res. 1999;39(2):113–23. https://doi.org/10.1006/phrs.1998.0413.
12. Koskela HO. Cold air-provoked respiratory symptoms: the mechanisms and management. Int J Circumpolar Health. 2007;66(2):91–100.
13. Sampson AP. The role of eosinophils and neutrophils in inflammation. Clin Exp Allergy. 2000;30(Suppl 1):22–7.
14. Parsons JP, Hallstrand TS, Mastronarde JG, Kaminsky DA, Rundell KW, Hull JH, et al. An official American Thoracic Society clinical practice guideline: exercise-induced bronchoconstriction. Am J Respir Crit Care Med. 2013;187(9):1016–27. https://doi.org/10.1164/rccm.201303-0437ST.

15. Maeda H, Nakagawa M, Yokoyama M. Hospital admissions for respiratory diseases in the aftermath of the great Hanshin earthquake. Nihon Kyobu Shikkan Gakkai Zasshi. 1996;34(2):164–73.
16. Nakazawa T, Kawakami Y, Sudo M, Kobayashi S, Suetsugu S, Nakajima S, et al. Asthma death among adults in Japan 1995–1997. Analysis of 295 cases reported questionnaires sent to hospitals with more than 100 beds. Asthma Death Investigation Committee. Arerugi. 2000;49(6):505–11.
17. Nakazawa T, Dobashi K. Current asthma deaths among adults in Japan. Allergol Int. 2004;53:205–9.
18. Fan F, Long K, Zhou Y, Zheng Y, Liu X. Longitudinal trajectories of post-traumatic stress disorder symptoms among adolescents after the Wenchuan earthquake in China. Psychol Med. 2015;45(13):2885–96. https://doi.org/10.1017/S0033291715000884.
19. Sakuma A, Takahashi Y, Ueda I, Sato H, Katsura M, Abe M, et al. Post-traumatic stress disorder and depression prevalence and associated risk factors among local disaster relief and reconstruction workers fourteen months after the Great East Japan Earthquake: a cross-sectional study. BMC Psychiatry. 2015;15:58. https://doi.org/10.1186/s12888-015-0440-y.
20. Tsutsui T, Hasegawa Y, Hiraga M, Ishiki M, Asukai N. Distinctiveness of prolonged grief disorder symptoms among survivors of the Great East Japan Earthquake and Tsunami. Psychiatry Res. 2014;217(1–2):67–71. https://doi.org/10.1016/j.psychres.2014.03.001.
21. Sandberg S, McCann DC, Ahola S, Oja H, Paton JY, McGuinness D. Positive experiences and the relationship between stress and asthma in children. Acta Paediatr. 2002;91(2):152–8.
22. Huovinen E, Kaprio J, Koskenvuo M. Asthma in relation to personality traits, life satisfaction, and stress: a prospective study among 11,000 adults. Allergy. 2001;56(10):971–7.
23. Ritz T, Steptoe A. Emotion and pulmonary function in asthma: reactivity in the field and relationship with laboratory induction of emotion. Psychosom Med. 2000;62(6):808–15.
24. Isenberg SA, Lehrer PM, Hochron S. The effects of suggestion and emotional arousal on pulmonary function in asthma: a review and a hypothesis regarding vagal mediation. Psychosom Med. 1992;54(2):192–216.
25. Liu LY, Coe CL, Swenson CA, Kelly EA, Kita H, Busse WW. School examinations enhance airway inflammation to antigen challenge. Am J Respir Crit Care Med. 2002;165(8):1062–7. https://doi.org/10.1164/ajrccm.165.8.2109065.
26. Hasegawa T, Koya T, Sakagami T, Muramatsu Y, Muramatsu K, Kagamu H, et al. Analysis of depression in asthmatic patients using the Japanese version of Patient Health Questionnaire-9. Allergol Int. 2012;61(3):475–87. https://doi.org/10.2332/allergolint.11-OA-0413.
27. Toyama M, Hasegawa T, Sakagami T, Koya T, Hayashi M, Kagamu H, et al. Depression's influence on the Asthma Control Test, Japanese version. Allergol Int. 2014;63(4):587–94. https://doi.org/10.2332/allergolint.14-OA-0708.
28. Elenkov IJ, Chrousos GP. Stress hormones, proinflammatory and antiinflammatory cytokines, and autoimmunity. Ann N Y Acad Sci. 2002;966:290–303.
29. Centers for Disease, Control Prevention (CDC). Self-reported increase in asthma severity after the September 11 attacks on the World Trade Center—Manhattan, New York, 2001. MMWR Morb Mortal Wkly Rep. 2002;51(35):781–4.
30. Brackbill RM, Hadler JL, DiGrande L, Ekenga CC, Farfel MR, Friedman S, et al. Asthma and posttraumatic stress symptoms 5 to 6 years following exposure to the World Trade Center terrorist attack. JAMA. 2009;302(5):502–16. https://doi.org/10.1001/jama.2009.1121.
31. Wisnivesky JP, Teitelbaum SL, Todd AC, Boffetta P, Crane M, Crowley L, et al. Persistence of multiple illnesses in World Trade Center rescue and recovery workers: a cohort study. Lancet. 2011;378(9794):888–97. https://doi.org/10.1016/S0140-6736(11)61180-X.
32. Mindlis I, Morales-Raveendran E, Goodman E, Xu K, Vila-Castelar C, Keller K, et al. Posttraumatic stress disorder dimensions and asthma morbidity in World Trade Center rescue and recovery workers. J Asthma. 2017;54(7):723–31. https://doi.org/10.1080/02770903.2016.1263650.

33. Fukuhara A, Sato S, Uematsu M, Misa K, Nikaido T, Inokoshi Y, et al. Impacts of the 3/11 disaster in Fukushima on asthma control. Am J Respir Crit Care Med. 2012;186(12):1309–10. https://doi.org/10.1164/ajrccm.186.12.1309.
34. Jentzsch NS, Camargos P, Sarinho ES, Bousquet J. Adherence rate to beclomethasone dipropionate and the level of asthma control. Respir Med. 2012;106(3):338–43. https://doi.org/10.1016/j.rmed.2011.12.001.
35. Marceau C, Lemiere C, Berbiche D, Perreault S, Blais L. Persistence, adherence, and effectiveness of combination therapy among adult patients with asthma. J Allergy Clin Immunol. 2006;118(3):574–81. https://doi.org/10.1016/j.jaci.2006.06.034.
36. Zheng S, Yu Q, Zeng X, Sun W, Sun Y, Li M. The influence of inhaled corticosteroid discontinuation in children with well-controlled asthma. Medicine (Baltimore). 2017;96(35):e7848. https://doi.org/10.1097/MD.0000000000007848.
37. Koyanagi K, Koya T, Sasagawa M, Hasegawa T, Suzuki E, Arakawa M, et al. An analysis of factors that exacerbate asthma, based on a Japanese questionnaire. Allergol Int. 2009;58(4):519–27. https://doi.org/10.2332/allergolint.09-OA-0095.
38. Japanese Society of Allergology. Risk factor of asthma. In: Asthma Prevention and Management Guideline 2006 (in Japanese). Tokyo, Japan: Japanese Society of Allergology; 2006. p. 29–41.

Chapter 6
Exacerbation of COPD by Air Pollution, Cold Temperatures, or Discontinuation of Medicine: What Should Be Measured to Help Prevent It?

Seiichi Kobayashi

Abstract Chronic obstructive pulmonary disease (COPD), which is a chronic lung disease characterized by airflow limitation, has become a major global public health problem. Natural disasters have a negative impact on the clinical outcomes of patients with COPD in the affected area. Hospital admissions for COPD exacerbations increase after a disaster and continue to increase for up to a month after the disaster. Due to power outages and equipment damage, patients with severe COPD receiving oxygen therapy have to find refuge in hospitals. Exposure to air pollution, including particulate matter and biological materials from the destruction of buildings and tsunami sludge, may contribute to the worsening of respiratory symptoms in patients with COPD. In the aftermath of a disaster, patients may lose their prescribed drugs and oxygen supplies or may be unable to access medical services, resulting in an increase in exacerbations. Patients may be exposed to cold temperatures in damaged houses or emergency shelters with insufficient fuel supplies and power failure and experience shortages of water, food, and sanitary goods, which may lead to poor personal hygiene. An outbreak of acute respiratory infections becomes a major concern. The unfavorable conditions are likely to result in the increased occurrence of exacerbations. Disaster preparedness for COPD patients should be considered before it becomes an emergency.

Keywords Chronic obstructive pulmonary disease (COPD) · Disaster · Exacerbation

---

S. Kobayashi
Department of Respiratory Medicine, Japanese Red Cross Ishinomaki Hospital, Ishinomaki, Japan
e-mail: skoba-thk@umin.ac.jp

K. Fujimoto (ed.), *Disaster and Respiratory Diseases*,
Respiratory Disease Series: Diagnostic Tools and Disease Managements,
https://doi.org/10.1007/978-981-13-2598-4_6

6.1 Introduction

Chronic obstructive pulmonary disease (COPD) is a common, preventable, and treatable disease that is characterized by persistent respiratory symptoms and airflow limitation due to airway and/or alveolar abnormalities usually caused by a significant exposure to noxious particles or gases, such as tobacco smoke [1]. Due to its increasingly high prevalence and associated morbidity and mortality, COPD has become a major global public health problem. Dyspnea, cough, and/or sputum production are the most frequent symptoms of COPD. COPD may be punctuated by an acute worsening of respiratory symptoms, called exacerbations. Exacerbations are important events in the management of COPD because they negatively impact the clinical status of the patients, rates of hospitalization and readmission, and disease progression.

Natural disasters, such as floods, hurricanes, volcanic eruptions, earthquakes, and tsunamis destroy buildings and vital infrastructure; they cause many deaths and traumatic injuries. In the aftermath of a disaster, sanitary conditions, medical resources, and public health services are also impaired. Survivors are exposed to air pollution, such as dust from a destroyed building. Under these conditions, patients with COPD are susceptible to an aggravation of their symptoms.

This article aims to review the evidence on exacerbation of COPD after natural disasters and discuss disaster preparedness for COPD patients.

6.2 Documented Issues for Patients with COPD

Several reports have documented exacerbations of COPD after natural disasters [2–5].

According to the reports from a regional core hospital in the affected area of the Great East Japan Earthquake disaster in 2011, admissions for COPD exacerbations increased after the disaster (Fig. 6.1) [3, 4]; the increase in exacerbations continued for up to 5 weeks after the disaster (Fig. 6.2) [4]. Patients with COPD showed greater physical inactivity than they did before the disaster [4].

Long-term oxygen therapy is prescribed for COPD patients with severe resting chronic hypoxemia. Several reports have documented that patients undergoing oxygen therapy evacuated to a healthcare facility after disasters, such as during the New York City Blackout in 2003 [6]; the three Hurricanes of Charley, Frances, and

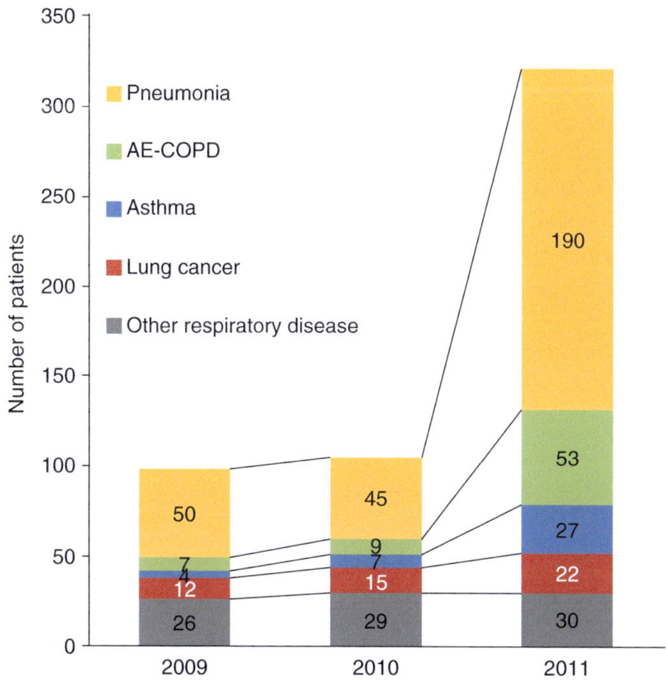

Fig. 6.1 Number and proportion of patients hospitalized for respiratory diseases, pooled from 11 March to 9 May in 2009, 2010, and 2011 at a regional core hospital in the affected area of the Great East Japan Earthquake disaster. AE-COPD, exacerbation of chronic obstructive pulmonary disease. Adapted from "The impact of the 2011 Great East Japan Earthquake on hospitalisation for respiratory disease in a rapidly aging society: a retrospective descriptive and cross-sectional study at the disaster base hospital in Ishinomaki," by Yamanda S, Hanagama M, Kobayashi S, Satou H, Tokuda S, Niu K, Yanai M, 2013, *BMJ Open, 3*, pii: e000865, doi: https://doi.org/10.1136/bmjopen-2012-000865, available under the Creative Commons Attribution-noncommercial License

Jeanne in 2004 [7]; and the Great East Japan Earthquake in 2011 [8, 9]. In Japan, after the Great Hanshin Earthquake of 1995, medical personnel and home oxygen therapy (HOT) service providers established emergency operation measures for a disaster, including a real-time patient locating system that was developed by the providers [8]. In the areas affected by the tsunami after the Great East Japan Earthquake, patients receiving oxygen therapy lost their stable oxygen supplies following power outage or equipment damage; oxygen providers did not have immediate access to the patients, and thus, oxygen-dependent patients presented to the hospital as "HOT refugees" (Fig. 6.3) [4, 8].

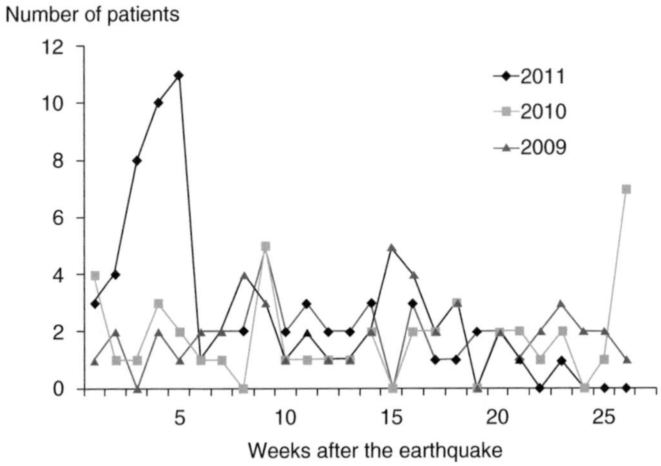

Fig. 6.2 Number of hospitalized patients with exacerbations of chronic obstructive pulmonary diseases at a regional core hospital in the affected area 6 months after the Great East Japan Earthquake disaster in 2011 and the corresponding periods in 2009 and 2010. Adapted from "Impact of a large-scale natural disaster on patients with chronic obstructive pulmonary disease: the aftermath of the 2011 Great East Japan Earthquake," by Kobayashi S, Hanagama M, Yamanda S, Satoh H, Tokuda S, Kobayashi M, Ueda S, Suzuki S, Yanai M, 2013, *Respir Investig, 51,* p. 17–23, doi: https://doi.org/10.1016/j.resinv.2012.10.004, available under the Creative Commons Attribution-noncommercial License

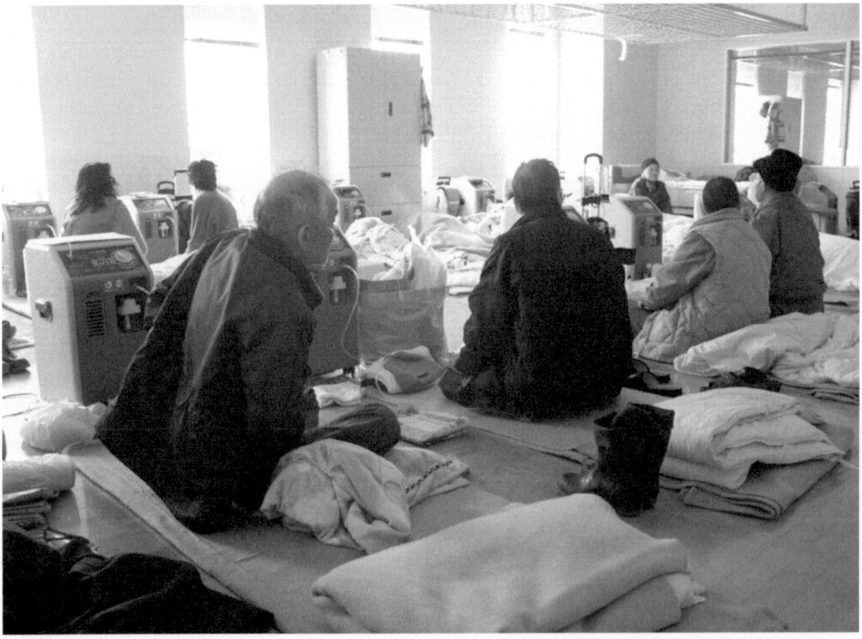

Fig. 6.3 A temporary shelter for patients needing oxygen therapy was established inside a regional core hospital in the affected area after the Great East Japan Earthquake in 2011. Adapted from "Home oxygen therapy during natural disasters: lessons from the great East Japan earthquake," by Kobayashi S, Hanagama M, Yamanda S, Yanai M, 2012, *Eur Respir J, 39*, p. 1047–8, doi: https://doi.org/10.1183/09031936.00149111. Copyright 2012 by the European Respiratory Society

Few guidelines for the management of COPD include a documented plan for emergency and disaster preparedness. There is no description of emergencies or preparedness for disasters in the Global Strategy for the Diagnosis, Management, and Prevention of Chronic Obstructive Lung Disease (GOLD) report [1], the Clinical Practice Guideline from the American College of Physicians, American College of Chest Physicians, American Thoracic Society (ATS), the European Respiratory Society (ERS) in 2011 [10], the official ERS/ATS Clinical Practice Guidelines in 2017 [11], and the UK National Institute for Health and Care Excellence (NICE) clinical guideline published in 2010 [12]. The Japanese Respiratory Society Guidelines for the Diagnosis and Treatment of COPD (chronic obstructive pulmonary disease) 4th edition, which was published in 2013, describe disaster preparedness based on the experience of the Great East Japan Earthquake in 2011.

6.3 Causes of COPD Exacerbations After Natural Disaster

COPD exacerbations are heterogeneous events caused by complex interactions between the host, respiratory pathogens, environmental pollutions, and other factors, leading to an increase in airway inflammation. The possible causes of exacerbations after a natural disaster are summarized in Table 6.1.

6.3.1 Respiratory Infections

Respiratory tract infections, either viral or bacterial or a combination of both, are the most important triggers of exacerbation [13, 14]. The common predominant bacteria from the lower airways of patients with COPD exacerbations are *Haemophilus influenzae*, *Streptococcus pneumoniae*, and *Moraxella catarrhalis* [15]. Patients with COPD often have bacteria colonizing their lower airway during

Table 6.1 Causes of COPD exacerbations after a natural disaster

Respiratory infections
Viruses
Bacteria
Atypical pathogens
Environmental factors
Air pollutions (dust and sludge)
Ambient temperature
Tobacco smoke
Medical loss and disaster-driven evacuation
Host factors
Poor mental health (anxiety and depression)
Physical inactivity

the stable phase of the disease. However, exacerbations are often associated with the isolation of new strains of airway bacteria, with an accompanying host inflammatory response to these new strains. Respiratory viruses, such as the influenza virus, parainfluenza virus, adenovirus, and rhinovirus, are most commonly involved in exacerbations [16]. Respiratory bacteria and viruses often act together, and coinfections can exert a synergistic inflammatory effect. Prevalence of these pathogens was reported to be significantly different in different locations, although there were diagnostic limitations in the microbiological tests.

Acute respiratory infections commonly occur after disasters [3]. However, little is known about the respiratory pathogens in exacerbations of COPD after disasters. After the Great East Japan Earthquake in 2011, outbreaks of influenza were reported in some evacuation centers [17, 18]; however, the increase in infection due to multiple-drug-resistant bacteria was not observed [19, 20]. COPD patients hospitalized with exacerbations were treated based on the consensus guidelines, without any problems, in areas affected by the Great East Japan Earthquake disaster [4]. Multiple-drug-resistant pathogens may not be common among patients without previous antimicrobial treatment or immunosuppressive therapy, even during disasters.

6.3.2 Environmental Factors

Exposure to air pollutants, including ozone (O_3), carbon monoxide (CO), nitrogen dioxide (NO_2), sulfur dioxide (SO_2), and particulate matters ($PM_{2.5}$, PM_{10}), has been associated with the risk of exacerbation [21, 22]. After a disaster, the concentrations of air pollutants are high in the affected areas [23]. Inhalation of dust from destroyed buildings [24] or tsunami sludge [25] is reported to be associated with a decreased lung function and onset of lung injury.

After the 2011 Great East Japan Earthquake following a tsunami, many buildings were destroyed, and the tsunami-affected area was covered by a thick layer of mud and debris. The tsunami sludge dried up and was scattered, thus acting as an air pollutant. In Ishinomaki, a port town located in northeast (Tohoku) Japan and one of the areas most affected by the Great East Japan Earthquake and tsunami, evacuees in emergency shelters complained of cough between late March and early April [26]. Hospital admissions due to the exacerbation of COPD increased during that period [4]. Particulate matters and biological materials from debris and tsunami sludge may have contributed to the worsening of respiratory symptoms among patients in the affected area.

A lower ambient temperature and winter season can lead to exacerbations of COPD [27, 28]. Cold temperatures are related to a reduction in lung function and immunity toward respiratory infections. Exposure to cold air can induce bronchoconstriction and decreased mucociliary clearance. COPD exacerbations are more common in the winter season when there are more respiratory viral infections prevalent in the community. After the 2011 Great East Japan Earthquake, patients were exposed to cold temperatures in damaged houses or emergency shelters with insufficient fuel supplies and power failure. Such unfavorable conditions are likely to result in the increased occurrence of exacerbations [4, 8].

6.3.3 Medication Loss and Disaster-Driven Evacuation

After a large-scale disaster, the continuity of routine medical care is challenging. Normal function is affected in healthcare facilities. Patients may lose their prescribed drugs and oxygen supplies or may be unable to access medical services. Maintenance therapy in COPD, such as smoking cessation, bronchodilators, rehabilitation, and vaccination, reduce the risk and frequency of exacerbations [1]. Interruption of regular treatment may result in an increase in COPD exacerbations [4].

In addition, disaster-driven evacuation itself may be associated with the risk of exacerbation. These conditions, in addition to insufficient fuel supplies, power failures, water and food shortages, and a lack of sanitary goods, result in poor personal hygiene. Such living conditions following the disaster likely reduce the oral health of almost all evacuees. Impairment of the swallow reflex, even without dysphagia, is observed in patients suffered from COPD exacerbations [29]; thus, patients with inadequate oral health may be silently aspirating bacteria-containing oropharyngeal or gastric secretions. The poor oral status of an evacuee is a potential risk factor for exacerbation. This is supported by the observation that fewer remaining teeth, a large amount of plaque, and a decreased frequency of teeth brushing are significantly correlated with COPD exacerbation [30].

6.3.4 Host Factors

Anxiety and depression are important comorbidities in patients with COPD; it is suggested that they carry an increased risk of exacerbations [31]. Natural disasters can have a negative impact on the mental and behavioral health, inducing anxiety, depression, and post-traumatic stress disorder (PTSD) in survivors [32], which may be a potential risk factor for COPD exacerbation.

The level of physical activity in a patient with COPD is associated with mortality and exacerbations [33]. It was previously reported that physical disability was an independent risk factor for death after the Hanshin-Awaji Earthquake [34] and the 1999 Taiwan Earthquake [35]. Those reports investigated mortality in the acute phase, but not hospitalizations during the subacute phases. After the Great East Japan Earthquake, patients who had a poor level of physical activity had an increased number of hospitalizations [4]. After the earthquake and tsunami, over 40,000 evacuees stayed in the crowded emergency shelters in Ishinomaki, where they had to sleep on the floor without beds. Elderly patients with COPD were largely sedentary, which led them to become physically inactive.

6.4 Prevention Measures for Exacerbation After Disasters

6.4.1 For Healthcare Providers

Patients with COPD should continue their medications during the disaster. Pharmacological therapy is used to reduce symptoms, improve exercise tolerance and health status, and reduce the frequency and severity of exacerbations [1]. Long-acting muscarinic antagonists (LAMAs) and long-acting β_2-agonists (LABAs) significantly improve lung function, dyspnea, and health status and reduce exacerbation rates. The effect of LAMAs on reducing exacerbations is greater than that of the LABAs. They also decreased hospitalizations. In patients with moderate to very severe COPD and exacerbations, an inhaled corticosteroid (ICS) combined with an LABA is more effective in improving lung function and health status of the patient and reducing exacerbations, than either component alone. However, regular treatment with ICSs increases the risk of pneumonia, especially in those with severe disease. Combination treatment with LABA and LAMA improves lung function and reduces symptoms more effectively than monotherapy. Moreover, treatment with LABA/LAMA reduces exacerbations more effectively than monotherapy or ICS/LABA. Triple inhaled therapy of ICS/LAMA/LABA improves lung function, symptoms, and health status and reduces exacerbations more effectively than ICS/LABA or LAMA monotherapy. A phosphodiesterase-4 inhibitor reduces moderate and severe exacerbations in patients with chronic bronchitis, severe to very severe COPD, and a history of exacerbations treated with systemic corticosteroids. Long-term azithromycin and erythromycin therapy are reported to reduce exacerbations in patients prone to exacerbations. Regular use of *N*-acetylcystein and carbocysteine may reduce the risk of exacerbations in select populations.

Keeping essential medications on hand at all times, rather than storing them at home, is recommended. Written summaries of health and medication information should be provided to patients in paper or in an electronic format. After the Great East Japan Earthquake in 2011, patient medication notebooks, which are provided by the registered Japanese health insurance pharmacies and have all prescriptions recorded, were reportedly useful in identifying regular medications [8].

Influenza vaccination reduces the total number of exacerbations and mortality and is recommended for all patients with COPD [1]. The pneumococcal vaccinations, pneumococcal conjugate vaccine (PCV13) and pneumococcal polysaccharide vaccine (PPSV23), are recommended for all patients older than 65 years of age. PPSV23 is also recommended for younger patients with COPD having significant comorbid conditions, including chronic heart or lung disease.

Management of COPD is not limited to pharmacological treatments and should be complemented by the appropriate pharmacological interventions. Patients with COPD should be educated about their disease and available treatments, including smoking cessation, improving exercise and physical activity levels, proper nutrition, medical adherence, correct use of inhaler devices, and coping skills. Self-management for good practice is essential in the management of COPD.

Education and self-management of diseases in regular times is useful for ensuring continuation of good behaviors after a disaster. After the Great East Japan Earthquake, patients who had enrolled in the Ishinomaki COPD Network (ICON), which is a regional medical liaison system aimed at the comprehensive care of patients with COPD in Ishinomaki and surrounding cities, continued good practice with exercise, writing a self-management diary, and adherence to prescribed inhalants, even when they evacuated to shelters. Over 90% of the patients continued their smoking cessation. A COPD action plan for emergency and disaster preparedness may be effective in reducing the risk of disease exacerbation during disasters.

The long-term administration of oxygen to patients with chronic respiratory failure increases the survival of patients with severe resting hypoxemia [1]. For patients undergoing oxygen therapy, it is recommended that they arrange for spare oxygen cylinders in case of electricity blackouts and that they plan for evacuating to a healthcare facility [8].

6.4.2 *For Disaster Relief Operations Personnel and Policy Makers*

Recent disasters, especially those in developed countries, have highlighted the importance of preparedness measures for noncommunicable diseases, including cardiovascular disease, cancers, diabetes, and chronic lung diseases. In the affected area of the Great East Japan Earthquake in 2011, a number of survivors reportedly experienced exacerbations of chronic illnesses due to the direct stress of the disaster, the interruption of care, or both. In this context, disaster medicine and preparedness should be based on a more comprehensive approach rather than on the traditional, injury-oriented approach.

A stable supply of essential drugs, in addition to psychological support, is important for maintaining disease control during a disaster. To achieve effective and efficient distribution of medications and medical supplies, a centralized organization for the coordination of distribution and receipt of healthcare resources is recommended. After the Great East Japan Earthquake, in Ishinomaki and the surrounding cities, medical relief teams rounded community evacuation centers and prescribed medications for patients with chronic disease [36]. These efforts minimized the interruption of treatment during the chronic phase.

Following devastating natural disasters, the threat of infectious disease outbreak becomes a major concern. Infection control measures are essential among survivors in community evacuation shelters [37].

The region's primary medical center is prepared for "HOT refugees" who require oxygen therapy. Community-based plans for patients receiving home oxygen therapy are also considered. In Ishinomaki, which is the area affected by the 2011 Great East Japan Earthquake, local governments, local medical associations, a regional core hospital, and home oxygen service providers agreed upon a system of preparedness for the HOT patients during a large-scale natural disaster in March 2017.

Older patients with COPD may consider evacuating from the areas affected by the disaster, because long periods in emergency shelters can result in deterioration in activity of daily living and hospitalization for exacerbations [3].

6.5 Conclusions

Natural disasters have a negative impact on the clinical outcomes of patients with COPD. Disaster preparedness for COPD patients in the affected area should be considered before the disaster. A stable supply of prescribed drugs and oxygen, in addition to psychological support, is essential to maintain disease control during a disaster. Avoiding exposure to air pollution prevents the worsening of respiratory symptoms. Favorable conditions of the necessities of life decrease the risk of exacerbations.

Respiratory physicians, in cooperation with disaster specialists, should develop strategies for the management of patients with COPD after natural disasters.

References

1. Global Initiative for Chronic Obstructive Lung Disease (GOLD). Global Strategy for the Diagnosis, Management and Prevention of COPD. 2017. http://www.goldcopd.org. Accessed 14 Dec 2017.
2. Ishihara K, Fujii H, Watanabe I, Hajiro T, Nishimura T, Okazaki M, et al. The Kobe earthquake and pulmonary disease. Kokyu. 1996;15:93–8. (in Japanese)
3. Yamanda S, Hanagama M, Kobayashi S, Satou H, Tokuda S, Niu K, et al. The impact of the 2011 Great East Japan Earthquake on hospitalisation for respiratory disease in a rapidly aging society: a retrospective descriptive and cross-sectional study at the disaster base hospital in Ishinomaki. BMJ Open. 2013;3. pii: e000865 https://doi.org/10.1136/bmjopen-2012-000865.
4. Kobayashi S, Hanagama M, Yamanda S, Satoh H, Tokuda S, Kobayashi M, et al. Impact of a large-scale natural disaster on patients with chronic obstructive pulmonary disease: the aftermath of the 2011 Great East Japan Earthquake. Respir Investig. 2013;51:17–23. https://doi.org/10.1016/j.resinv.2012.10.004.
5. Ohkouchi S, Shibuya R, Yanai M, Kikuchi Y, Ichinose M, Nukiwa T. Deterioration in regional health status after the acute phase of a great disaster: respiratory physicians' experiences of the Great East Japan Earthquake. Respir Investig. 2013;51:50–5. https://doi.org/10.1016/j.resinv.2012.12.003.
6. Prezant DJ, Clair J, Belyaev S, Alleyne D, Banauch GI, Davitt M, et al. Effects of the August 2003 blackout on the New York City healthcare delivery system: a lesson for disaster preparedness. Crit Care Med. 2005;33:S96–101.
7. Platz E, Cooper HP, Silvestri S, Siebert CF. The impact of a series of hurricanes on the visits to two central Florida Emergency Departments. J Emerg Med. 2007;33:39–46.
8. Kobayashi S, Hanagama M, Yamanda S, Yanai M. Home oxygen therapy during natural disasters: lessons from the great East Japan earthquake. Eur Respir J. 2012;39:1047–8. https://doi.org/10.1183/09031936.00149111.

9. Sato K, Morita R, Tsukamoto K, Sato N, Sasaki Y, Asano M, et al. Questionnaire survey on the continuity of home oxygen therapy after a disaster with power outages. Respir Investig. 2013;51:9–16. https://doi.org/10.1016/j.resinv.2012.10.005.
10. Qaseem A, Wilt TJ, Weinberger SE, Hanania NA, Criner G, van der Molen T, et al. Diagnosis and management of stable chronic obstructive pulmonary disease: a clinical practice guideline update from the American College of Physicians, American College of Chest Physicians, American Thoracic Society, and European Respiratory Society. Ann Intern Med. 2011;155:179–91. https://doi.org/10.7326/0003-4819-155-3-201108020-00008.
11. Wedzicha JA, Calverley PM, Albert RK, Anzueto A, Criner GJ, Hurst JR, et al. Prevention of COPD exacerbations: a European Respiratory Society/American Thoracic Society guideline. Eur Respir J. 2017;50:16002265. https://doi.org/10.1183/13993003.02265-2016.
12. National Institute for Health and Care Excellence. Chronic obstructive pulmonary disease in over 16s. 2010. http://www.nice.org.uk/guidance/cg101. Accessed 14 Dec 2017.
13. Wedzicha JA, Seemungal TA. COPD exacerbations: defining their cause and prevention. Lancet. 2007;370:786–96. https://doi.org/10.1016/S0140-6736(07)61382-8.
14. Celli BR, Barnes PJ. Exacerbations of chronic obstructive pulmonary disease. Eur Respir J. 2007;29:1224–38. https://doi.org/10.1183/09031936.00109906.
15. Sethi S, Murphy TF. Infection in the pathogenesis and course of chronic obstructive pulmonary disease. N Engl J Med. 2008;359:2355–65. https://doi.org/10.1056/NEJMra0800353.
16. Mohan A, Chandra S, Agarwal D, Guleria R, Broor S, Gaur B, et al. Prevalence of viral infection detected by PCR and RT-PCR in patients with acute exacerbation of COPD: a systematic review. Respirology. 2010;15:536–42. https://doi.org/10.1111/j.1440-1843.2010.01722.x.
17. Hatta M, Endo S, Tokuda K, Kunishima H, Arai K, Yano H, et al. Post-tsunami outbreaks of influenza in evacuation centers in Miyagi Prefecture. Jpn Clin Infect Dis. 2012;54:e5–7. https://doi.org/10.1093/cid/cir752.
18. Kamigaki T, Seino J, Tohma K, Nukiwa-Soma N, Otani K, Oshitani H. Investigation of an Influenza A (H3N2) outbreak in evacuation centres following the Great East Japan earthquake, 2011. BMC Public Health. 2014;14:34. https://doi.org/10.1186/1471-2458-14-34.
19. Takahashi H, Fujimura S, Ubukata S, Sato E, Shoji M, Utagawa M, et al. Pneumonia after Earthquake, Japan, 2011. Emerg Infect Dis. 2012;18:1909–11. https://doi.org/10.3201/eid1811.111660.
20. Aoyagi T, Yamada M, Kunishima H, Tokuda K, Yano H, Ishibashi N, et al. Characteristics of infectious diseases in hospitalized patients during the early phase after the 2011 great East Japan earthquake: pneumonia as a significant reason for hospital care. Chest. 2013;143:349–56. https://doi.org/10.1378/chest.11-3298.
21. Sint T, Donohue JF, Ghio AJ. Ambient air pollution particles and the acute exacerbation of chronic obstructive pulmonary disease. Inhal Toxicol. 2008;20:25–9. https://doi.org/10.1080/08958370701758759.
22. Li J, Sun S, Tang R, Qiu H, Huang Q, Mason TG, et al. Major air pollutants and risk of COPD exacerbations: a systematic review and meta-analysis. Int J Chron Obstruct Pulmon Dis. 2016;11:3079–91. https://doi.org/10.2147/COPD.S122282. eCollection 2016
23. Yamamoto R, Nagai N, Koizumi N, Ninomiya R. Dust concentration around the sites of demolition work after the Great Hanshin-Awaji Earthquake. Environ Health Prev Med. 1999;3:207–14.
24. Aldrich TK, Gustave J, Hall CB, Cohen HW, Webber MP, Zeig-Owens R, et al. Lung function in rescue workers at the World Trade Center after 7 years. N Engl J Med. 2010;362:1263–72. https://doi.org/10.1056/NEJMoa0910087.
25. Yamanda S, Kobayashi S, Hanagama M, Sato H, Suzuki S, Ueda S, et al. Two cases of tsunami dust pneumonia: organizing pneumonia caused by the inhalation of dried tsunami sludge after the 2011 Great East Japan Earthquake. Intern Med. 2016;55:3645–53. https://doi.org/10.2169/internalmedicine.55.6952.

26. Yanai M, Kobayashi S, Hanagama M, Yamanda S, Satoh H. Respiratory diseases related to a tsunami disaster. Nihon Naika Gakkai Zasshi. 2012;6:1727–35. https://doi.org/10.2169/naika.101.1727. (in Japanese)
27. Tseng CM, Chen YT, Ou SM, Hsiao YH, Li SY, Wang SJ, et al. The effect of cold temperature on increased exacerbation of chronic obstructive pulmonary disease: a nationwide study. PLoS One. 2013;8:e57066. https://doi.org/10.1371/journal.pone.0057066.
28. Donaldson GC, Goldring JJ, Wedzicha JA. Influence of season on exacerbation characteristics in patients with COPD. Chest. 2012;141:94–100. https://doi.org/10.1378/chest.11-0281.
29. Kobayashi S, Kubo H, Yanai M. Impairment of the swallowing reflex in exacerbations of COPD. Thorax. 2007;62:1017. https://doi.org/10.1136/thx.2007.084715.
30. Liu Z, Zhang W, Zhang J, Zhou X, Zhang L, Song Y, et al. Oral hygiene, periodontal health and chronic obstructive pulmonary disease exacerbations. J Clin Periodontol. 2012;39:45–52. https://doi.org/10.1111/j.1600-051X.2011.01808.x.
31. Laurin C, Moullec G, Bacon SL, Lavoie KL. Impact of anxiety and depression on chronic obstructive pulmonary disease exacerbation risk. Am J Respir Crit Care Med. 2012;185:918–23. https://doi.org/10.1164/rccm.201105-0939PP.
32. Goldmann E, Galea S. Mental health consequences of disasters. Annu Rev Public Health. 2014;35:169–83. https://doi.org/10.1146/annurev-publhealth-032013-182435.
33. Garcia-Aymerich J, Lange P, Benet M, Schnohr P, Anto JM. Regular physical activity reduces hospital admission and mortality in chronic obstructive pulmonary disease: a population based cohort study. Thorax. 2006;61:772–8. https://doi.org/10.1136/thx.2006.060145.
34. Osaki Y, Minowa M. Factors associated with earthquake death in the great Hanshin-Awaji earthquake. Am J Epidemiol. 1995;153:153–6.
35. Chou YJ, Huang N, Lee CH, Tsai SL, Chen LS, Chang HJ. Who is at risk of death in an earthquake? Am J Epidemiol. 2004;160:688–95. https://doi.org/10.1093/aje/kwh270.
36. Ishii T. Medical response to the Great East Japan Earthquake in Ishinomaki City. Western Pac Surveill Response J. 2011;2:10–6. https://doi.org/10.5365/WPSAR.2011.2.4.005.
37. Centers for Disease Control and Prevention. Infection Control Guidance for Community Evacuation Centers Following Disasters. http://www.cdc.gov/disasters/commshelters.html. Accessed 14 Dec 2017.

Chapter 7
Onset of DVT or Pulmonary Thromboembolism Related to the Life in a Car or Narrow Shelter: What Should We Do to Prevent the Onset of the Pulmonary Thromboembolism?

Kazuhiko Hanzawa

Abstract Pulmonary embolism occurred frequently after Mid Niigata Prefecture Earthquake and Kumamoto Earthquake due to car shelter. Many calf DVTs have been detected in these areas after earthquake. It has been reported that calf DVT causes fatal pulmonary embolism. Car shelter had been demonstrated to be related with calf DVT in Kumamoto Earthquake. Also, since many people evacuated into their own car after Emilia Earthquake in Italy, many DVTs were detected 2 years after the earthquake, and a woman died from pulmonary embolism during car shelter. Therefore, car shelter after earthquake clearly relates with calf DVT and pulmonary embolism.

Keywords Pulmonary embolism · DVT · Earthquake · Car shelter

7.1 Introduction

Pulmonary embolism occurred frequently after Mid Niigata Prefecture Earthquake and Kumamoto Earthquake, and deaths from it were reported. We have studied deep vein thrombosis (DVT) in some quake area residents for 14 years. I would like to discuss about pulmonary embolism and DVT after earthquake.

Pulmonary embolism after earthquake first received attention after the Mid Niigata Prefecture Earthquake in 2004. Many aftershocks occurred following the Mid Niigata Prefecture Earthquake. The number of shelter was limited. As a result, up to around 50,000 people stayed inside their cars parked next to their houses as a

---

K. Hanzawa
Advanced Treatment and Prevention for Vascular Disease and Embolism,
Niigata University Graduate School of Medicine and Dental Sciences, Niigata, Japan

K. Fujimoto (ed.), *Disaster and Respiratory Diseases*,
Respiratory Disease Series: Diagnostic Tools and Disease Managements,
https://doi.org/10.1007/978-981-13-2598-4_7

temporary shelter (Fig. 7.1). In addition, in order to save gasoline and avoid cold, people appeared to have continued to evacuate into own small compact cars with narrow seats for both family members and pets. As a result, pulmonary embolism occurred frequently, and many people experienced sudden death. According to our investigation, 11 people determined symptomatic pulmonary embolism in 2 weeks after the earthquake, and 6 of them died. Moreover, all six fatal cases were women younger than 50 years (Fig. 7.2).

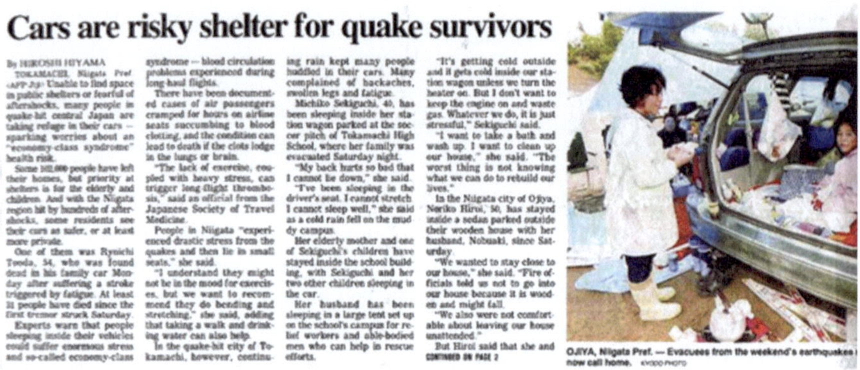

Cars are risky shelter for quake survivors

By HIROSHI HIYAMA

TOKAMACHI, Niigata Pref. (AFP-Jiji) Unable to find space in public shelters or fearful of aftershocks, many people in quake-hit central Japan are taking refuge in their cars — sparking worries about an "economy-class syndrome" health risk.

Some 102,000 people have left their homes, but priority at shelters is for the elderly and children. And with the Niigata region hit by hundreds of aftershocks, some residents see their cars as safer, or at least more private.

One of them was Ryuichi Tooda, 34, who was found dead in his family car Monday after suffering a stroke triggered by fatigue. At least 31 people have died since the first tremor struck Saturday.

Experts warn that people sleeping inside their vehicles could suffer enormous stress and so-called economy-class syndrome — blood circulation problems experienced during long-haul flights.

There have been documented cases of air passengers cramped for hours on airline seats succumbing to blood clotting, and the condition can lead to death if the clots lodge in the lungs or brain.

"The lack of exercise, coupled with heavy stress, can trigger long-flight thrombosis," said an official from the Japanese Society of Travel Medicine.

People in Niigata "experienced drastic stress from the quakes and then lie in small seats," she said.

"I understand they might not be in the mood for exercises, but we want to recommend they do bending and stretching," she said, adding that taking a walk and drinking water can also help.

In the quake-hit city of Tokamachi, however, continuing rain kept many people huddled in their cars. Many complained of backaches, swollen legs and fatigue.

Michiko Sekiguchi, 40, has been sleeping inside her station wagon parked at the soccer pitch of Tokamachi High School, where her family was evacuated Saturday night.

"My back hurts so bad that I cannot lie down," she said.

"I've been sleeping in the driver's seat. I cannot stretch. I cannot sleep well," she said as a cold rain fell on the muddy campus.

Her elderly mother and one of Sekiguchi's children have stayed inside the school building, with Sekiguchi and her two other children sleeping in the car.

Her husband has been sleeping in a large tent set up on the school's campus for relief workers and able-bodied men who can help in rescue efforts.

"It's getting cold outside and it gets cold inside our station wagon unless we turn the heater on. But I don't want to keep the engine on and waste gas. Whatever we do, it is just stressful," Sekiguchi said.

"I want to take a bath and wash up. I want to clean up our house," she said. "The worst thing is not knowing what we can do to rebuild our lives."

In the Niigata city of Ojiya, Noriko Hiroi, 50, has stayed inside a sedan parked outside their wooden house with her husband, Nobuaki, since Saturday.

"We wanted to stay close to our house," she said. "Fire officials told us not to go into our house because it is wooden and might fall.

"We also were not comfortable about leaving our house unattended."

But Hiroi said that she and

CONTINUED ON PAGE 2

OJIYA, Niigata Pref. — Evacuees from the weekend's earthquakes now call home. KYODO PHOTO

Fig. 7.1 Car shelter risky shelter for quake survivors (from the Japan Times)

Symptomatic pulmonary embolism in car shelter after Mid Niigata Earthquake 2004

Age/ gender	Car shelder (day)	Type of car	Position of seat	On set after quake	Prognosis	Tranquilizer	Walking bathroom
79/F	14	Sedan	Rear	2 w	Alive	No	+
76/F	2	Sedan	Rear	2 d	Alive	+	+
75/F	3	Unknown	Unknown	7 d	Alive	Unknown	Unknown
64/F	5	Unknown	Unknown	5 d	Alive	Unknown	Unknown
60/F	14	Sedan	Rear	2 w	Alive	No	+
50/F	6	Small car	Unknown	6 d	Dead	+	No
50/F	2	Unknown	Unknown	2 d	Dead	Unknown	Unknown
48/F	5	Wagon	Front	5 d	Dead	+	No
47/F	5	Unknown	Unknown	5 d	Dead	Unknown	No
46/F	2	Unknown	Unknown	6 d	Dead	Unknown	Unknown
43/F	4	Small car	Rear	4 d	Dead	+	No

Fig. 7.2 Symptomatic pulmonary embolism after Mid Niigata Prefecture Earthquake

Ro et al. conducted autopsies of Japanese people who died of pulmonary embolism outside of hospitals in 2003 and demonstrated that blood clot formed in the soleus muscle vein was pathologically responsible for pulmonary embolism [1]. Thus, lower extremity deep vein thrombosis was recognized as the cause of pulmonary embolism in Japan (this has previously been well-recognized in western countries). Furthermore, Ro et al. provided evidence that more than 90% of fatal pulmonary embolisms outside of hospital were induced by repeated thrombi [2]. Chronic-repeated thrombi suddenly became larger after the attachment of new thrombi. Accordingly, in order to prevent pulmonary embolism, detection of organic thrombi (old thrombi) is also important. Moreover, Ogi et al. reported that thrombi were more likely to be formed in a larger diameter soleus vein (7 mm or larger), and the individual was more susceptible to pulmonary embolism [3]. Since many individuals preferred car shelters (about 50,000 people at day 10 in Mid Niigata Prefecture Earthquake), it was assumed that an intervention would be needed because of the potentially high frequency of thrombi developing in the soleus muscle among individuals in disaster areas. We used portable ultrasound machine and screened thrombi in calf vein at the disaster areas. Standard ultrasonographic examination of the lower extremity veins is conducted on the femoral vein. However, as described above, since pulmonary embolisms that occur outside of the hospital are caused by thrombi located in the soleus muscles in the lower legs, screening was conducted only for the veins in the lower legs, in a sitting position (Fig.7.3). Moreover, the maximum diameter of the soleus muscle was also measured. This

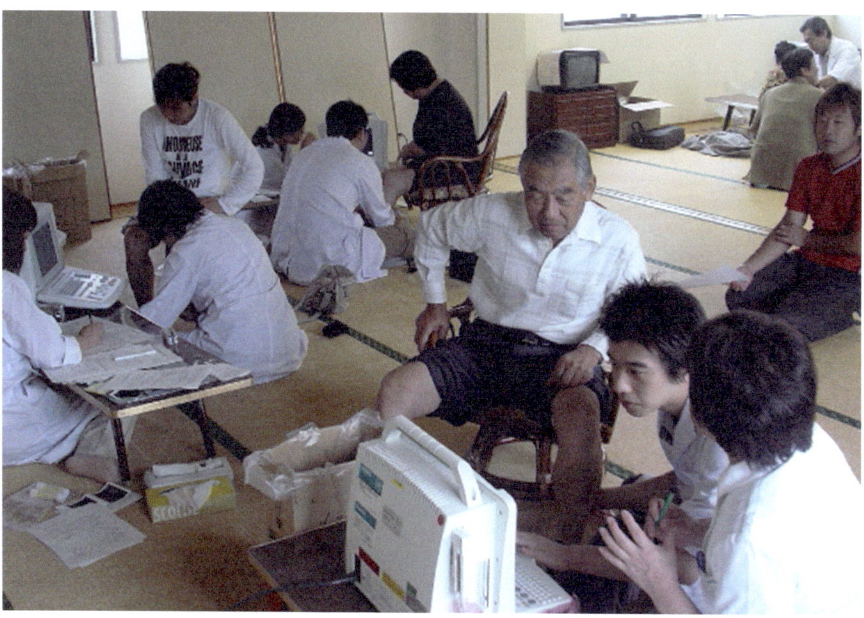

Fig. 7.3 Screening for thrombus in lower legs by ultrasound (Mid Niigata Prefecture Earthquake)

method is called the "Chuetsu method," and it was utilized during the Niigataken Chuetsu-oki Earthquake and Iwate-Miyagi Nairiku Earthquake, the Emilia Earthquake, and Kumamoto Earthquake.

After the Mid Niigata Prefecture Earthquake, screening for the prevention of pulmonary embolism was conducted for more than 1 year after the earthquake. Many deep vein thrombosis (DVT) cases were detected in the legs. Accordingly, in March 2006, through collaboration among the Niigata Prefecture, Niigata Medical Association, and Niigata University, screening for the prevention of economy class syndrome was conducted among residents at Aga town in Niigata Prefecture, using the Chuetsu method. It was treated as screening at an earthquake control area. As a result, the incidence of DVT at disaster areas after the Mid Niigata Prefecture Earthquake in October and November 2005 was 7.8%, while it was 1.8% in Aga town, significantly lower. Accordingly, DVT that was detected 1 year or later after the earthquake was demonstrated to be related to the natural disaster. Therefore, again through collaboration among the Niigata Prefecture, Niigata Medical Association, and Niigata University, "Diagnosis and Treatment Guidelines for Deep Vein Thrombosis (DVT)/Pulmonary Embolism (PE) after the Mid Niigata Prefecture Earthquake" was prepared to help manage DVT at hospitals in disaster areas (Fig. 7.4). According to the Guideline, when a thrombus is detected in the soleus vein by ultrasonography, D-dimer blood test should be conducted. If it is within 2× of the reference range, the subject should be instructed to wear graduated elastic

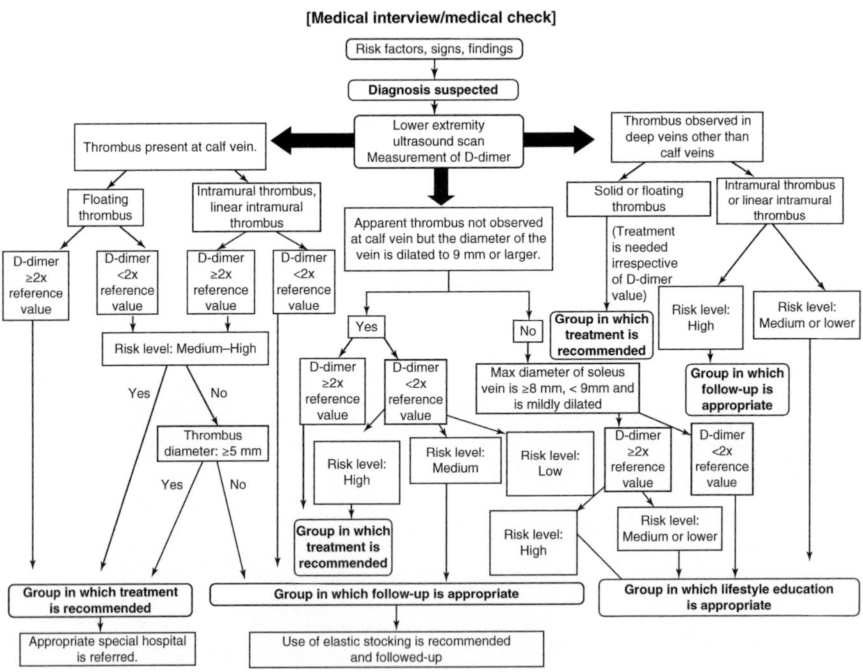

Fig. 7.4 Diagnosis and treatment guideline for deep vein thrombosis

stocking (for treatment) and be given lifestyle guidance. If the value is higher than 2× of the reference range, the subject should receive a medical check-up at a medical institution, and pharmacotherapy should be provided. This Guideline was utilized since August 2006 and has been used as a screening method to prevent economy class syndrome after the Noto Earthquake in 2007, Niigata-Ken Chuetsu-oki Earthquake in 2007, Iwate-Miyagi Nairiku Earthquake in 2008, Great East Japan Earthquake in 2011, and Northern Italy Earthquake in 2012. We continue to conduct screening at disaster areas after the Mid Niigata Prefecture Earthquake but still detect DVT at an incidence of 6–7%, which is higher than that for control areas (Fig. 7.5).

We elucidate whether asymptomatic calf DVT induced pulmonary embolism 8 years after Mid Niigata Prefecture Earthquake. Subjects were 1419 residents in the area of Mid Niigata Prefecture Earthquake (Ojiya city and Tokamachi city). Calf DVT was determined by compression ultrasound examination. Six residents had pulmonary embolism, and 31 residents had IS after the quake. The positive rate of pulmonary embolism (3.3%) in the residents with calf DVT was significantly higher than that in those without it (0.13%) (Odds ratio = 7.84 $p < 0.0001$). Most calf DVT occurred after the quake may induce pulmonary embolism.

7.1.1 DVT After Emilia Earthquake in Italy

A series of epicentral earthquakes occurred at Emilia-Romagna, Modena, near Bologna in northern Italy from May through June 2012 (the Emilia Earthquake). We visited the local area to investigate refugee sites a month after the earthquake. There were many refugee camps at the struck areas, and portable beds were installed. However, as the investigation proceeded, it was revealed that more than 20,000

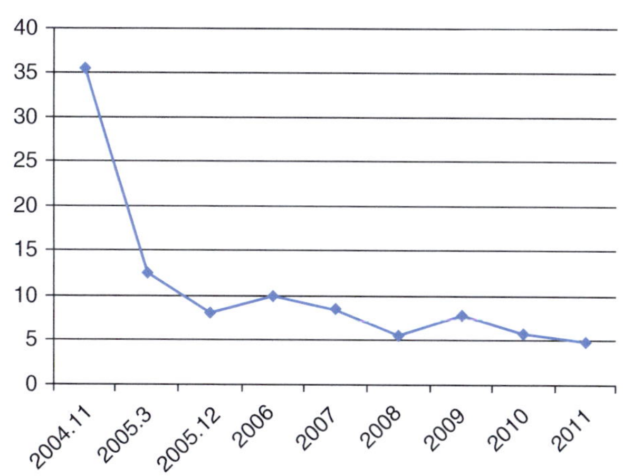

Fig. 7.5 Positive rate of calf DVT in the area of Mid Niigata Prefecture Earthquake since 2004

people were not at refugee sites, but at preferred car shelters (Fig. 7.6). In addition, the incidence of DVT and pulmonary embolism had increased after the earthquake (Fig. 7.7). Eventually, one woman who used a car shelter died from pulmonary embolism.

This situation was quite similar to that after the Mid Niigata Prefecture Earthquake. Accordingly, because of the potential increase of DVT, after various arrangements, we have conducted prevention efforts for pulmonary embolism using the Chuetsu method since March 2013 (Fig. 7.8). For 1 year after April 2013, it was financially supported by Niigata Prefecture Earthquake Recovery Fund. With sup-

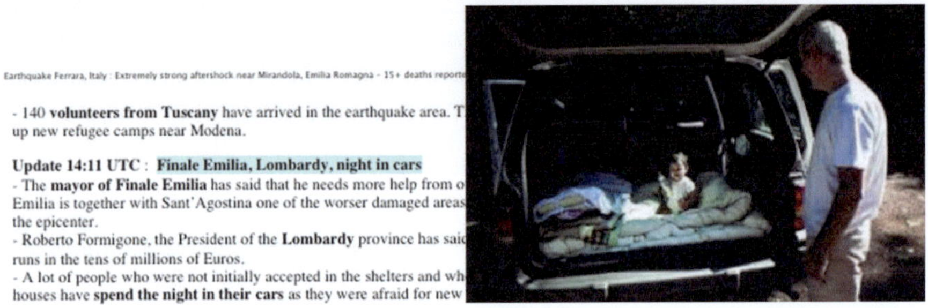

Fig. 7.6 Car shelter in Finale Emilia 2012

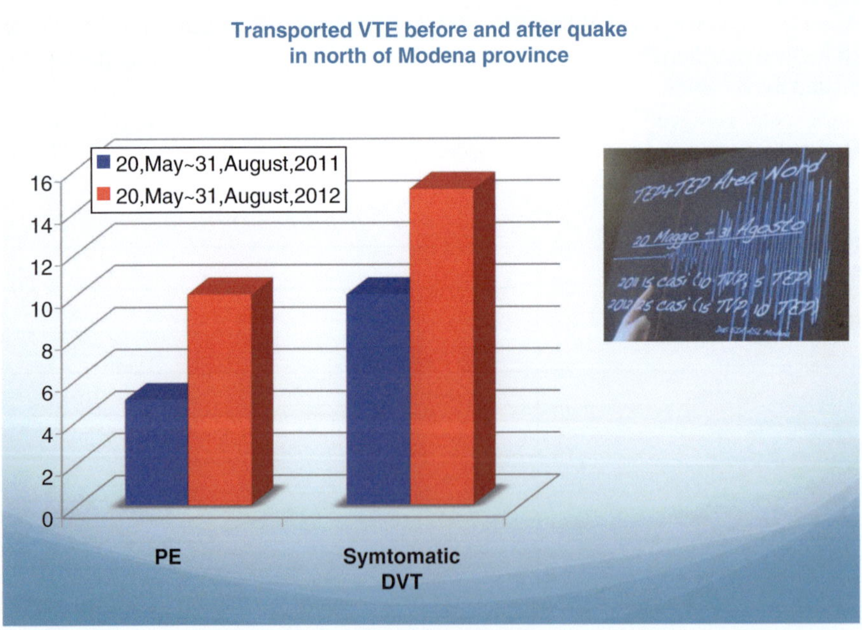

Fig. 7.7 DVT/PE before and after Emilia Earthquake (Modena University)

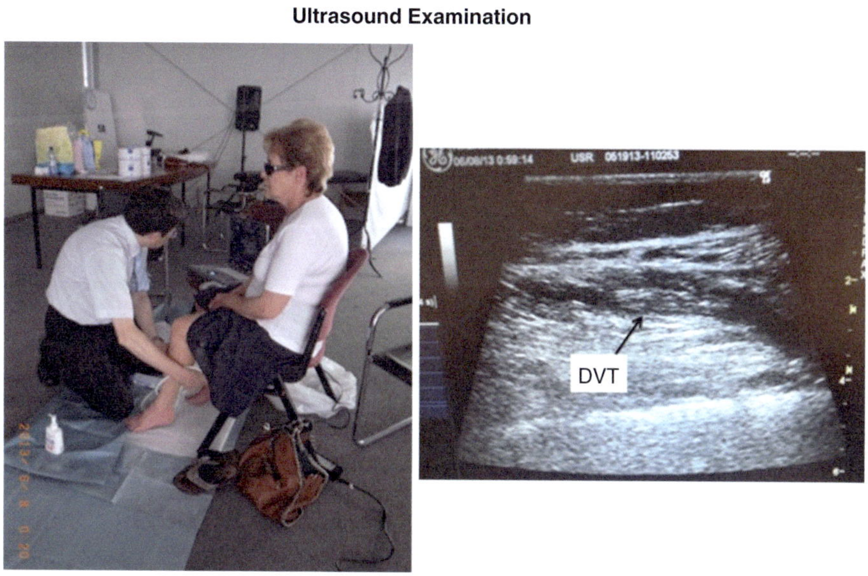

Fig. 7.8 Screening for calf DVT by ultrasound (the Chuetsu method) in Modena

port from local Italian doctors and volunteers, screening was conducted at Finale Emilia, Cavezzo, Mirandola, Concordia, Guastalla, Modena, San Felice sul Panaro, Caripi, and Soliera until November 2014. In addition, in September and October 2014, screening was conducted at Trento, as a control site for the Italian Earthquake.

As a result, a total of 447 people were screened at Emilia Earthquake refugee areas. Among them, DVT was detected in 49 people (11%). At a control city and Trento, 52 people were screened, and DVT was observed in 2 (3.8%). DVT was seen in people in their 30s and older, and it was higher than the age distribution of the DVT incidence in the US (Fig. 7.9).

After L'Aquila Earthquake in 2009, with collaboration with Professor Ferri and Professor Grassi at the Department of Cardiovascular Diseases and Nephrology at the University of L'Aquila, we have conducted screening based on the Chuetsu method from April 2014 through February 2016. Among 111 residents at L'Aquila, DVT was detected in 7 (6.3%). Accordingly, at Modena province where the earthquake occurred, the incidence of DVT is about 2.8 times higher even 1 year after the earthquake. In addition, it was still 1.7 times higher in L'Aquila even 5 years after the earthquake. This suggests that DVT is still preventable in Italy even when a significant time has elapsed after the earthquake. Unfortunately, pulmonary embolism frequently occurred after Kumamoto Earthquake in 2016. After Kumamoto Earthquake, water, electricity, and gas supply were stopped for a few days. And logistics stopped by some reason. Therefore, many people had dehydration state after the earthquake due to shortage of foods and drinks. People are scared of aftershock and evacuated into their own small car, because roof of houses or buildings might fall. These situations induced econ-

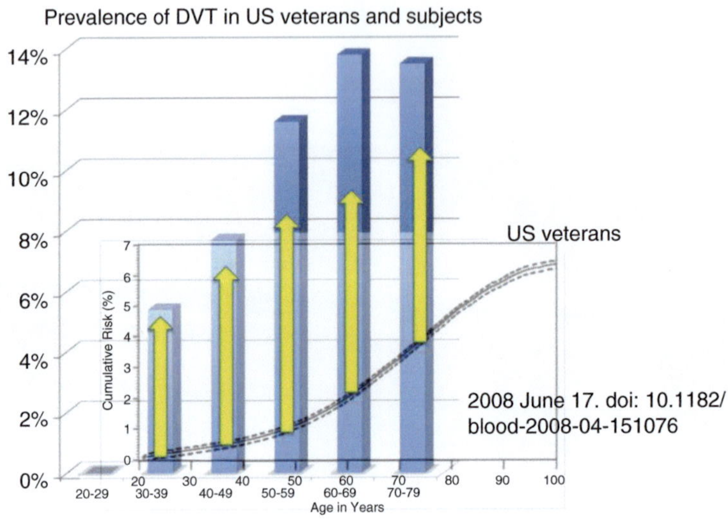

Fig. 7.9 Comparison of prevalence of DVT in US veterans and residents in Emilia Earthquake

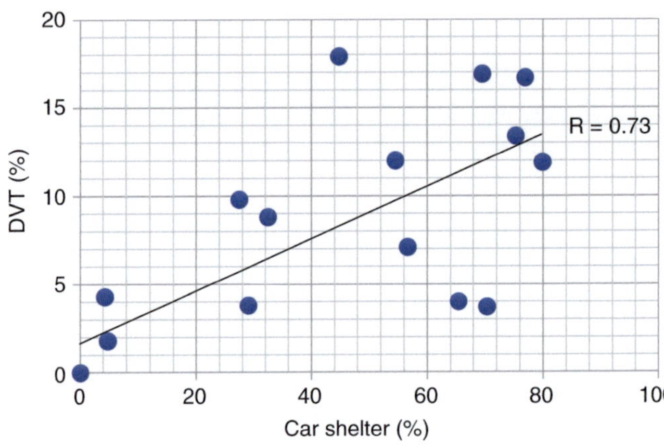

Fig. 7.10 Relationship between frequency of car shelter and calf DVT in 17 evacuation facilities 3 weeks after Kumamoto Earthquake

omy class syndrome. More than ten severe acute pulmonary embolisms were transported to hospital during 2 days after the earthquake due to car shelter. 51 years old woman died from pulmonary embolism during car shelter. We attempted to check-up calf DVT by compression ultrasound examination for calf vein to prevent pulmonary embolism in Kumamoto city 3 weeks after the earthquake. Subjected were 993 evacuees in 17 public evacuation facilities. Figure 7.10 shows correlation between the positive rate of calf DVT in evacuee and that of car shelter experience after the earthquake. Therefore, car shelter is clearly an important risk factor for DVT and pulmonary embolism (Fig. 7.10).

7.2 Conclusion

Car shelter after earthquake is clearly a cause of pulmonary embolism. We should prepare for enough shelter after natural disaster including earthquake. Because people evacuate into their own car if the space of shelter was narrow or parivacy could not be maintained. We also remember that DVT after earthquake have a possibility of pulmonary embolism.

References

1. Ro A, Kageyama N, Tanifuji T, Kobayashi M, Takada A, Murai T. Histopathological study of pulmonary arteries in 14 autopsy cases with massive pulmonary thromboembolism. Leg Med (Tokyo). 2003;(Supple 1):s315–7.
2. Ro A, Kageyama N. Clinical significance of the Soleal vein and related drainage veins, in calf vein thrombosis in autopsy cases with massive pulmonary thromboembolism. Ann Vasc Dis. 2016;(1):15–21.
3. Ohgi S, Tachibana M, Ikebuchi M, Kanaoka Y, Maeda T, Mori T. Pulmonary embolism in patients with isolated soleal vein thrombosis. Angiology. 1998;49(9):759–64.

Part III
Aggravation of Existing Respiratory Diseases by the Lack of Health Resource due to the Lifeline Stoppage

Chapter 8
What a Patient and His Family Should Do When Unable to Continue Home Oxygen Therapy and Home Mechanical Ventilation During a Blackout: When Unable to Continue Home Oxygen Therapy and Noninvasive Positive-Pressure Ventilation due to a Power Outage, What Should the Patient and Family Member(s) Do?

Fumi Nishizaki, Kazuo Kitou, and Satoshi Kuboike

Abstract A power outage triggered by a large-scale disaster deactivates medical devices used for in-home therapies, such as home oxygen therapy (HOT) and non-invasive positive-pressure ventilation (NPPV), rendering patients suddenly unable to continue their therapies. In this article, we mainly report the measures taken by home medical care service providers during past large-scale disasters to consider preparations for and actions to be taken during a disaster, such that patients and family members can continue in-home therapies. We also discuss the behaviors of patients and family members noted through their experiences, along with lessons learned, problems, and points to reflect upon. In Japan, there is a saying that goes, "Be prepared, and have no worries." We hope this article prompts patients and family members to consider or imagine a situation like "what would I do if a large-scale disaster strikes now and a power outage cuts off the oxygen supply?" and make the necessary preparations to protect themselves.

Keywords Great East Japan Earthquake · Preparations for disasters · D-MAP

F. Nishizaki (✉) · K. Kitou
Home Healthcare Sales Planning Department, Teijin Pharma Limited, Tokyo, Japan
e-mail: f.nishizaki@teijin.co.jp

S. Kuboike
Osaka Branch, Teijin Home Healthcare Limited, Kobe, Hyogo, Japan

K. Fujimoto (ed.), *Disaster and Respiratory Diseases*,
Respiratory Disease Series: Diagnostic Tools and Disease Managements,
https://doi.org/10.1007/978-981-13-2598-4_8

8.1 Introduction

Japan is a land of four distinct seasons filled with scenic beauty and abundant nature but is also one of the most seismically active nations in the world. Aside from earthquakes, the country is also subject to many types of natural disasters that can trigger power outages, such as typhoons, tsunamis, localized torrential rain, heavy snow, tornados, and volcanic eruptions.

Today, an estimated 170,000 patients receive home oxygen therapy (HOT) in Japan [1]. According to the results of a questionnaire survey targeting HOT/noninvasive positive-pressure ventilation (NPPV) patients, 52% of the respondents answered "power outages and disasters" as their "concerns and complaints that had arisen since the start of in-home therapies" [2]. In fact, each year, a large number of home-care patients and family members have been forced to evacuate because their home mechanical devices failed following an extensive power outage caused by a sudden disaster. To ensure that patients can feel at ease about undergoing in-home therapies in this country, where disaster-related power outages are frequent, it is extremely important for each of us to make appropriate preparations by learning what to prepare for beforehand and how to act once a disaster strikes, based on the lessons learned through our past experiences. To help home-care patients safely continue to undergo their HOT and noninvasive positive-pressure ventilation (NPPV) without any worries, this article explains how patients and family members should prepare for disasters, based on the reports of a home medical care service provider (hereinafter "service provider") experienced in actual disaster assistance operations.

8.2 History of Disaster Response: Evolving Disaster Response Measures

In Japan, HOT was approved for coverage under the National Health Insurance (NHI) in 1985, i.e., more than 30 years ago. In this section, we first explain the NHI system concerning in-home therapies in our country. When a doctor provides an in-home therapy for a patient, the following are specified as the requirements for the doctor to claim medical remuneration for "HOT instruction/management and supplies": "In case of lending medical device owned by an NHI-authorized medical institution (such as oxygen concentrators) to the patient, the NHI-authorized medical institution must provide sufficient maintenance and management services for the medical device. Should the services be entrusted to a service provider, the NHI-authorized medical institution must close a contract concerning the maintenance and management of the medical device with the service provider, explain details of the services to the patient, conduct periodic follow-ups and patient education, and ensure that the medical device continues to be serviced adequately by the service provider."

Under this NHI system, the patient rents a medical device for home use, such as an oxygen delivery device and NPPV device, from an NHI-authorized medical institution (hereinafter, "medical institution") and the maintenance/management of the rented device is provided by the medical institution or a service provider contracted by the medical institution. Furthermore, the "maintenance services for medical devices" outsourced by a medical institution encompass emergency response, and thus, service providers also offer aid in the event of a disaster.

Although service providers always try to stay in touch with communities and maintain close communication with patients, family members, and medical institutions, individual service providers build their own systems for medical device maintenance services and emergency response, and therefore, their services vary in content, quality, and scale.

As an example of the actions taken by these service providers, we now review the disaster response measures taken by Company A, a provider of home medical care services in Japan. Company A currently has about 100 sales offices nationwide and more than 1000 staff members dedicated to home medical care services. Since its inception in 1982, Company A has always considered that the essence of in-home therapy lies in patient-centered care. To provide "worry-free and reliable" medical care for patients in their own homes away from healthcare professionals, the company has aimed to offer 24/7 services all year around since before the time of cellular phones, and it has built a system that allows them to reach patients quickly in times of device malfunctions and power outages. This basic principle has remained unchanged to date, but their disaster response measures have continued to evolve with technological advancements and lessons learned from experiencing many disasters through more than 30 years of its history.

Company A overhauled their "Emergency Response Manual" based on their experience of delivering oxygen tanks to patients in the areas affected by power outages resulting from a severe storm during typhoon No. 19 in 1991 and formulated the "Typhoon Countermeasure Manual for Home Oxygen." Then, the Great Hanshin-Awaji Earthquake occurred in 1995. In addition to causing widespread power outages, it also severed roads, collapsed buildings, and triggered fires, resulting in a major disaster with a death toll exceeding 5000. Amid such devastation, Company A checked on the safety of patients and provided them with essential items such as oxygen concentrators and tanks despite difficult traffic conditions. Through this major earthquake disaster, Company A learned that medical institutions in the affected areas are so busy handling rapidly increasing numbers of injured people and inpatients, that service providers need to check on the safety of home-care patients receiving HOT or NPPV and report to the medical institutions. Additionally, they realized that service providers' sales offices in the affected areas are not sufficiently equipped to handle disasters of this magnitude due to limited human resources, supplies, and medical device, and thereby, they require backup from outside the affected areas. Based on this experience, Company A formulated the "Earthquake Disaster Countermeasure Manual for Home Medical Care." It is noteworthy that the manual specified the following: (1) "roles of the emergency headquarters and clarification of the intergroup collaboration system"; (2) "methods of communication and patient safety checks"; and (3) "the procedure for delivering oxygen tanks to patients." This manual has since been reviewed periodically, and the content and systems have been revised as needed. Additionally, the company has conducted trainings and disaster drills to promote the penetration of the manual's content among its employees. Furthermore, based on the lessons learned through experiencing major traffic congestion caused by destroyed or severed roads, the company has strengthened its system for the delivery of critical items by encouraging regional offices to apply for an emergency vehicle priority permit before a disaster.

During the Niigata Chuetsu Earthquake that occurred in 2004, power outages deactivated oxygen delivery devices, and the company reacknowledged that oxygen tanks were the only source of oxygen. They built additional stockpiling bases of oxygen tanks across the country and substantially increased their stockpiles. Subsequently, during the Niigata Chuetsu-oki Earthquake of 2007, many staff members were gathered from all over Japan for backup, and a large map was displayed on a wall at the local disaster countermeasure headquarter to map out the locations of patients, which turned out to be useful for collaborating with staff members who were unfamiliar with situations in local shelters and the local geography and enabled them to communicate with patients and medical institutions swiftly. This experience later led Company A to develop its own disaster response support map system called "Disaster Mapping Assistant Partner (D-MAP)," which has been put into practical use since October 2010.

The "D-MAP" is the electronic map information system developed by Company A using IT technologies to facilitate swift response even during an emergency (Fig. 8.1). Once the system receives information on an earthquake with an intensity of "5 lower" greater on the seven-point Japanese seismic scale, staff members are automatically notified via e-mail[*3] of the geographical extent of the affected areas

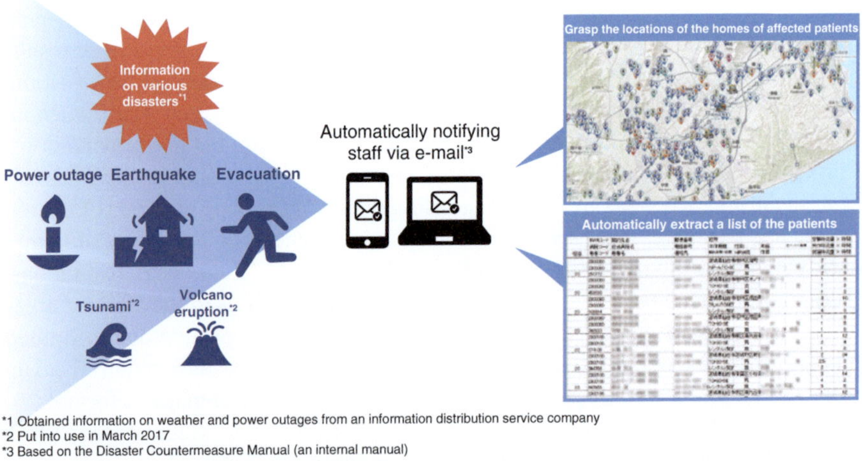

Fig. 8.1 Disaster mapping assistant partner (D-MAP) system

and number of affected people. The "D-MAP" shows the map of the affected areas and provides information on patients living there (the name, address, contact, secondary contact, device used, dose of oxygen prescribed, etc.), which allows staff members to grasp the situation at once. Furthermore, a list of the patients in the affected areas is automatically extracted, enabling staff members to quickly mobilize emergency response operations, including safety checks on patients and making arrangements for oxygen tanks.

Until now, Company A has experienced several disasters, and each time, they have strengthened their disaster preparedness capabilities both through software and hardware upgrades to ensure the timely provision of oxygen to patients (Fig. 8.2). However, when patients and family members cannot be reached, it hampers their support operations. Therefore, in the event of a disaster, patients and family members need to remain calm and secure their own safety first, and then notify service providers of their safety and locations, as quickly as possible, in order to continue receiving oxygen even at chaotic local shelters or medical institutions, or the places they have evacuated to outside the affected areas (a relative's house, hotel, etc.). First, they should contact their medical institutions to ask about how they or their contracted service providers are prepared for disasters and what disaster response measures they have taken in the past, and share multiple emergency contacts with them to receive timely assistance in case of a disaster.

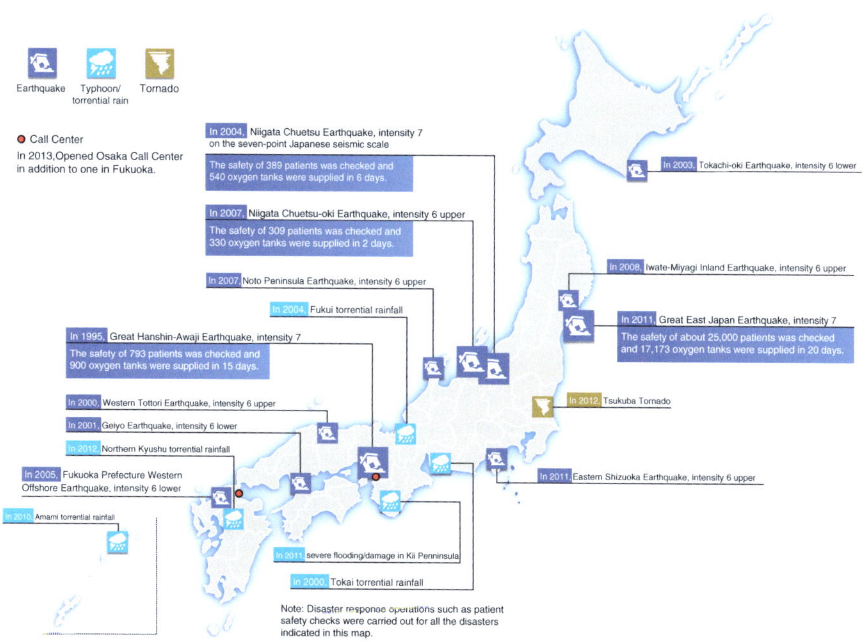

Fig. 8.2 Recent natural disasters in Japan (earthquakes, typhoons/torrential rains, tornadoes) and disaster assistance provided by Company A

8.2.1 Measures Taken During the Great East Japan Earthquake

At 2:46 p.m. on March 11, 2011, Japan was struck by the Great East Japan Earthquake, a magnitude 9.0 earthquake with a seismic intensity of 7, which also generated a massive tsunami with a maximum height of over 40 m, causing unprecedented damages. In this earthquake disaster, situations far worse than those assumed by the company A in its manuals occurred in succession, but their established systems and stockpiles functioned effectively (Table 8.1). Four minutes after the earthquake struck, Company A followed the manual mentioned before and established the disaster countermeasure headquarters in its Sendai branch and the disaster assistance headquarters in the Tokyo head office. Ten minutes after the quake, a list of approximately 25,000 patients living in the affected areas was extracted from the "D-MAP," and approximately 50 staff members at the disaster assistance headquarters started checking on the safety of each patient by telephone. As a Push Emergency Aid, the company also went forward with a plan to dispatch backup staff from all over Japan to the affected areas, and arranged emergency transportation of the essential items, such as oxygen concentrators and tanks, from their stockpiling warehouses located across the country. The number of patients who needed to be contacted for safety checks was 30 times higher than that during the Great Hanshin-Awaji Earthquake (approximately 800), but the company could contact about half of those patients in just 2 days, despite the extremely poor communication services. Once the attempt to contact patients by telephone had reached its limit, they started visiting patients' homes directly, while working with patients' associations to encourage the remaining patients to contact the service provider through television and other mass media outlets. As a result, Company A succeeded in checking the safety status of 98.8% of applicable patients in 2 weeks, and 99.8% by the end of March (in 3 weeks) (Fig. 8.3). During this process, it was useful to have patients' secondary emergency contacts on the D-MAP.

Additionally, when contacted by patients, overflowed calls to the sales offices in the affected areas were automatically transferred to the Fukuoka Call Center; this system worked effectively, resolving patients' concerns related to the inability to get calls through.

Regarding the transportation of essential items, Company A received cooperation from the affiliated freight company, along with the emergency vehicle priority permit mentioned before, and had more than 600 oxygen concentrators and more

Table 8.1 Comparison between the Great Hanshin-Awaji and Great East Japan Earthquakes

	Great Hanshin-Awaji Earthquake (1995)	Great East Japan Earthquake (2011)
Seismic intensity	7	7
Status of safety checks	793 patients in 15 days	About 25,000 patients in 20 days
Number of oxygen tanks supplied	900	17,173

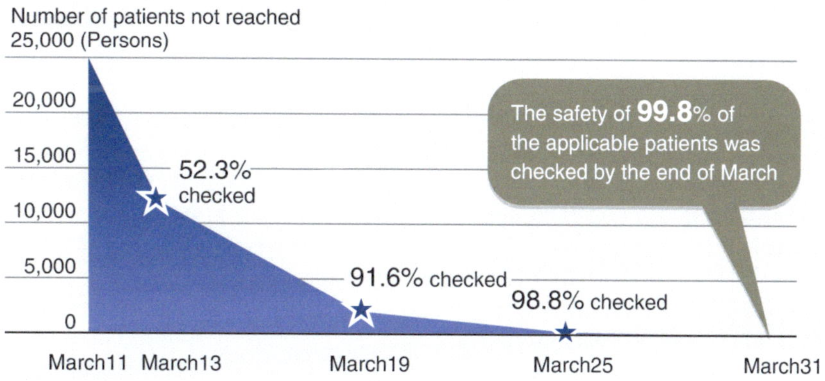

Fig. 8.3 Progress in safety checks on patients in all the affected areas during the Great East Japan Earthquake

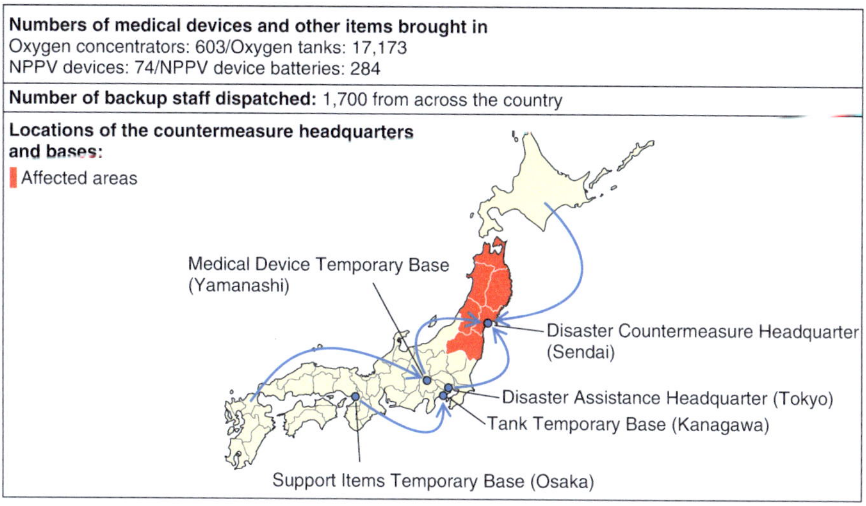

Fig. 8.4 Home medical care support provided by Company A during the Great East Japan Earthquake

than 17,000 oxygen tanks brought into the Tohoku region from all over Japan. In addition to patients' homes, many oxygen concentrators were placed at medical institutions and shelters to help setup temporary "HOT stations" to enable patients to continue their oxygen therapies. The number of staff members dispatched to the affected areas from other parts of Japan was approximately 40 per day, totaling 1700 by the end of June (Fig. 8.4).

Here, we describe the extensive power outages that occurred during the Great East Japan Earthquake and the rolling blackouts that were implemented subsequently. This earthquake disaster affected multiple power stations, including the Fukushima Daiichi Nuclear Power Station, as well as substations and transmission facilities, causing widespread power outages across eastern Japan. The power outages immediately after the earthquake were gradually resolved by the recovery efforts at power facilities, but restoration at the Fukushima Daiichi Nuclear Power Station was expected to take time. Therefore, 3 days after the disaster, rolling blackouts—a measure to ensure steady electricity supply—were implemented (the areas were divided into groups and electricity delivery to each group was stopped for approximately 2 h each day, in rotation, to reduce peak energy demand and to prevent prolonged power outage caused by a power shortage).

On the night of March 13, 2 days after the disaster, the implementation of rolling blackouts was hastily decided upon and the government requested service providers, including Company A, to contact all home-care patients in the affected areas. Therefore, staff members, except for those engaged in patient safety checks at the disaster assistance headquarter, started calling patients after 11 p.m. and were successful in contacting about 24,000 patients in the Kanto region by 6 a.m. next morning. Despite getting calls late at night, many patients said, "Thank you for contacting me," which was encouraging for the staff members. However, this episode also revealed that it is difficult for municipalities, medical institutions, and home-visit nursing facilities to make emergency contact with home-care patients, and that this can be done only by service providers.

Based on the lessons learned from their experiences in the Great East Japan Earthquake, Company A adopted some new measures. Immediately after the earthquake disaster, both cellular phones and landlines were flooded with a high volume of calls, making communication extremely difficult. Due to this experience, Company A installed battery-operated phones and line-powered phones at all of its sales offices. Additionally, to ensure that there will be no delay in checking on the safety of patients and communicating with medical institutions about disaster response measures, it installed satellite phones at all its branch offices, because they can provide coverage across extensive areas. The "D-MAP" was also improved by adding a feature that allows for real-time sharing of the information confirmed by sales offices away from disaster-struck areas via telephones. In 2015, another improvement was made to the "D-MAP" by incorporating information on power outages and evacuation (evacuation advisory and evacuation order announced by local municipalities) in addition to earthquake information. Additionally, Company A reacknowledged the importance of call centers as the liaison between patients and medical institutions. Particularly, when the implementation of rolling blackouts was announced, the phone lines were temporarily flooded with a sudden influx of orders for oxygen tanks from patients. Considering the possibility that the Fukuoka Call Center may get affected by a disaster, the company opened its second call center in Osaka, as a reinforcement measure against major disasters that can cause extensive damages.

8.2.2 Measures Taken During the Kumamoto Earthquakes

In April 2016, the Kumamoto Earthquakes struck with epicenters in Kumamoto Prefecture. In the foreshock (magnitude 6.5) on April 14, only two prefectures were considered affected according to the definition set by the Earthquake Disaster Countermeasure Manual, but the number of affected prefectures increased to seven after the main shock on April 16 (magnitude 7.3). Both quakes occurred during the night, and patients and their family members were forced to spend the night in pitch-black darkness due to a blackout, most likely, with tremendous anxiety. Following the foreshock, safety checks using the D-MAP were conducted with 90% of the 1241 applicable patients within 10 h, and they were completed in 22 h. After the mains hock, safety checks were conducted with 90% of the 3611 applicable patients within 12 h, and they were completed in 40 h (Fig. 8.5). When conducting the safety checks following the foreshock, staff members also confirmed patients' secondary contacts, which certainly helped in the safety checks after the mains hock. Company A had accumulated experiences through multiple disasters, strengthened their methods of communication as described before, increased their regional stockpiles of oxygen concentrators and tanks, and had staff members already experienced in disaster support operations across the country. All these factors contributed to their efficient oxygen delivery to patients both night and day.

To prepare for the next disaster, Company A added three more important features to the D-MAP based on the opinions and requests of staff members involved in the disaster support operations for Kumamoto Earthquakes, and the company upgraded its version in March 2017. The following features were included in the new version: (1) "Disaster simulation": To act calmly in the event of a disaster, this function allows staff members to know in advance which patients live in high-hazard areas by combining a hazard map and patient information so that they can set the priorities of safety checks and develop countermeasures through simulations ahead of a

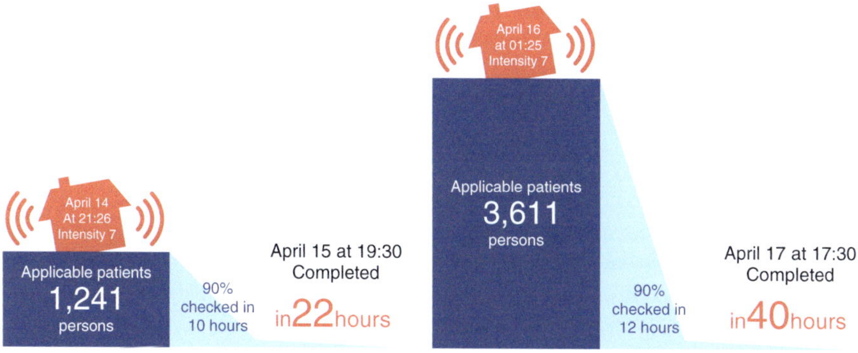

Fig. 8.5 Safety checks conducted during the 2016 Kumamoto Earthquakes

disaster. (2) "Facilitation of smooth information sharing": To support affected areas through companywide efforts, improvements were made so that disaster information is managed in a unified manner and is visualized. This made it possible to check on the safety of patients assigned to affected sales offices and to recover infrastructures such as phones and e-mail not just from the call centers but from all over the country. (3) "Compatibility with smartphones and tablets": Previously, the "D-MAP" was accessed only from PCs at sales offices, but the new feature allows staff members working in affected areas to use their cellular phones to directly access the system. With this, staff can now check the latest information on evacuation and power recovery in the field, thereby enabling them to respond more swiftly to patients and secure their own safety. Company A has also added information on tsunamis and volcanoes to the "D-MAP" system.

Aside from natural disasters, power outages continue to occur in some places in Japan daily due to sudden accidents, electrical constructions, etc. Based on the power outage information automatically distributed by the "D-MAP," staff members across the nation have been working on providing swift and detailed services for patients.

8.3 Limitations of Service Providers

Since the Great East Japan Earthquake, Company A has been working on enlightening the public by actively disclosing information through publication of academic papers and lecture presentations. Within the industry, the Japan Industrial and Medical Gases Association (JIMGA) streamlined the matters concerning emergency/disaster response systems, including specific procedures based on the lessons learned from how maintenance service providers for oxygen delivery devices had responded during the Great East Japan Earthquake and other disasters, so that patients can feel more at ease about undergoing HOT. In 2017, JIMGA published "Guidelines for Streamlining the Emergency/Disaster Response Systems for the Maintenance Service Providers for Home Oxygen Delivery Devices" [3] to improve the quality of maintenance services for home oxygen delivery devices in our country and to increase the efficiency of service providers as a whole, including small service providers.

In terms of the safety checks on patients, however, service providers carry them out based on individual contracts with medical institutions and thus cannot obtain information on patients outside their contract. Furthermore, to protect patients' privacy, patient information cannot be shared between service providers. To facilitate the quick and smooth rescue of patients, it is necessary for the government and local municipalities to take initiative in establishing "assistance networks for disaster emergency evacuation" at a national level.

Additionally, although HOT is provided according to the contract between a service provider and a medical institution, the costs of disaster response measures are generally not included in the contract. JIMGA's "agreement on the supply of medical gases and other related items in the time of a disaster" with prefectural governments specifies that the materials provided as instructed by a prefecture shall be settled later at reasonable prices at pre-disaster levels. We are requesting that this agreement be also applied to HOT so that service providers can settle the expenses required in their assistance operations after the disaster [4].

8.4 Development of Home Medical Devices

The top three improvements that patients seek in their home medical devices are "downsizing, portability/lightening, and low electricity consumption" for stationary oxygen concentrators and "portability/lightening, longer duration, and downsizing" for oxygen tanks. Additionally, the Ministry of Health, Labour and Welfare conducted a questionnaire survey targeting healthcare professionals in mostly home medical care support clinics and home-visit nursing stations as part of its "Project for Furthering the Approvals of Medical Devices to Promote In-home Medical Care" in 2013. According to the survey results published as "an investigative report on the needs for medical devices in in-home medical care," healthcare professionals also desired downsizing, lightening, and portability, as patients did. Additionally, they also expressed the needs for an oxygen concentrator that can switch to an oxygen tank during power outage, a remote control that can remotely switch flow rates, and an oxygen concentrator with voice guidance and/or indicator lights for elderly patients and patients with impaired vision or hearing disability [5]. Moreover, an increasing number of patients are living in "cluster housing such as care facilities," which has generated needs for a function to send an alarm to caretakers' rooms and transportable devices that can be moved from a bed room to a dining hall and other areas.

Patients have always requested "downsizing, lightening, energy saving, and longer duration," and service providers have continued working on developing improved devices. In case of Company A's oxygen concentrators, they have reduced the volume, weight, and energy usage by more than half in the last 15 years. Their oxygen tanks are no longer made of steel but are made of carbon fiber instead, which has cut the weight by about half. They have also developed oxygen tanks that can last three to four times longer than continuous-flow systems depending on the demand valve. A small, portable oxygen concentrator weighing less than 3 kg has also been developed, and it is currently used by some patients who require low flow oxygen. This portable oxygen concentrator contains an internal battery and can also be charged via car cigarette lighter, which helped some patients continue receiving oxygen by feeding power to their devices from cars during the Kumamoto Earthquakes. Other devices that have been developed include an oxygen concentrator that can automatically switch to an oxygen tank at the time of a power outage; an oxygen concentrator containing a battery to allow for more time to switch to an oxygen tank; and a remotely controllable oxygen concentrator with a universal design featuring audio guidance, indicator lights, and Braille displays for elderly users and those with disabilities. In terms of NPPV devices, "prolonged battery life" is also desired in addition to "downsizing," "portability/lightening," and "low energy consumption" and thus, service providers have worked on developing internal/external batteries for their devices. It is important for service providers to continue to be responsive to the needs of patients and healthcare professionals, along with changes in patients' living environments and technological advancements, and to predict disasters in the near future to develop better medical devices to provide for the society.

8.5 Conclusion: Disaster Response Through Mutual Support

To provide HOT with a greater sense of security, support from many doctors, nurses, and other healthcare professionals is important, and, for them to be able to collaborate with one another in a time of a disaster, it is essential that they are always prepared. After the Great East Japan Earthquake, a new section called "Disaster Response" was added to the Japanese Respiratory Society's 4th revised edition of Guidelines for the Diagnosis and Treatment of COPD (Chronic Obstructive Pulmonary Disease) (2013) and 2nd revised edition of Noninvasive Positive Pressure Ventilation (NPPV) Guidelines (2015) [6, 7]. Furthermore, the following statement has been added as a requirement to claim medical remuneration for "HOT instruction/management": "A doctor who ordered HOT must indicate the method of oxygen administration for HOT (the device, gas flow rate, duration of inhalation, etc.), emergency contact methods, and other instructions on the device, while explaining to the patient what to do in emergency situations including night-time emergency." Company A has created an information brochure called "Preparations for Disasters," [8] to supplement doctors' explanation to patients (Table 8.2). The "Preparations for Disasters" brochure describes what patients and family members can do to prepare for and to act appropriately during two types of situations; ordinary times and times of emergency. A major disaster causes extensive damages, stalling medical services, local municipalities, businesses, communication networks, and transportation and other infrastructures in the affected areas. Therefore, patients and family members should not forget that the concept of "self-help"—protecting themselves—is fundamental to disaster prevention. To act calmly without panicking during a disaster, it is important to be prepared in ordinary times. Patients should write down any information provided by the doctor, such as disease conditions, medications, and oxygen dose, on a medical record handbook or somewhere easy to find, and they should always carry this record/card with them/display it in a conspicuous place. It is also vital to prepare an oxygen tank and learn how to operate it, practice necessary breathing techniques such as pursed-lip breathing, prepare flash lights for power outages, and write down important emergency contact information. Furthermore, to receive aid from the community in addition to a service provider during a disaster, patients should go over the content of the "Disaster Evacuation Assistance System" of their local municipality ahead of a disaster, and they should register to ensure that

Table 8.2 The "Preparations for Disasters" brochure based on [8]

Preparing for a disaster	In the event of a disaster …
1. Check the contact information of the medical institution and HOT service provider • Display it in a conspicuous place • Carry the "Emergency Card" with you whenever you leave home	1. Secure your own safety and make sure that any source of fire is turned off • Watch out for falling furniture • Keep the oxygen tube away from an open flame
2. Check the name of your disease, medication(s), oxygen dose, and other important information • Use the "**Emergency Card**" to manage information • Consult your doctor about medication that you could take in case your physical condition deteriorates (during a disaster, you are more likely to have an acute exacerbation due to environmental degradation)	2. Switch to an oxygen tank (only if your doctor has instructed you to use an oxygen tank) • When your oxygen concentrator is deactivated due to a power outage or other reasons, switch to oxygen inhalation via the oxygen tank
3. Prepare the oxygen tank (only if your doctor has instructed you to use an oxygen tank) • Remember how many hours a single oxygen tank lasts • Frequently check how much oxygen is left and store the oxygen tanks in an easily accessible place • If you use a respiration-synchronized demand valve, keep extra batteries handy	3. Contact your HOT service provider • Contact your HOT service provider to receive adequate oxygen supply. There is a sticker indicating "Emergency Contacts" (the sales office in charge of your device and your local sales office) on your oxygen concentrator
4. Prepare a flash light and portable radio for power outages • To prepare for a sudden power outage, keep a flash light by your pillow and (or) in a room where you spend a lot of time • A portable radio is useful for obtaining information	4. If you evacuate your home, leave a note in a conspicuous place (such as by the front door), specifying where you will be moving to • The information would be helpful in determining where to send your oxygen delivery device

(continued)

Table 8.2 (continued)

Preparing for a disaster	In the event of a disaster …
5. Learn breathing techniques • It will help you feel relaxed and breathe efficiently 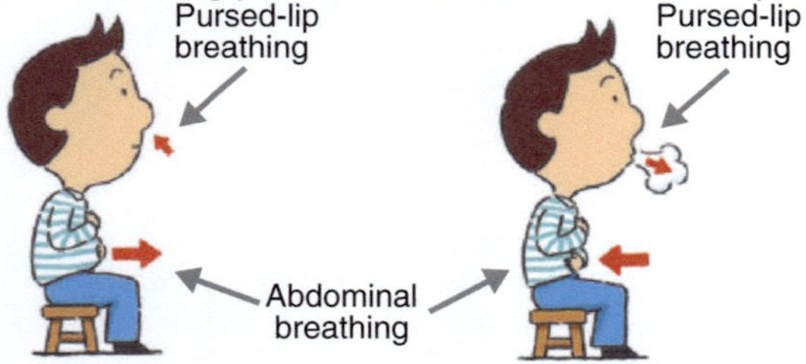 	
6. The support system for "people requiring evacuation assistance" • Check details of the system of your local municipality and consider utilizing it	
"Emergency Card" Contact Name: .... Primary contact: Phone: ...—...—... Secondary contact: Phone: ...—...—... (c/o) Shelter: .... Medical Institution: .... (Phone: — —) Primary care physician: Dept. ...... Dr. ...... Service provider: Contact: ...... Office Phone: ...—...—... Contact: ...... Office Phone: ...—...—...	Prescription Date: / / Disease: .... Medication(s): Medication(s) taken daily: .... Medication(s) taken when feeling ill: .... Oxygen inhalation volume (L/min) at rest, ... during activity, ... during sleep ...... Use of a NPPV device: Yes/No (Usage hours : - :) Other things to note: ....

their name is included in the list of people requiring evacuation assistance, which can bring peace of mind in the event of an emergency. Moreover, patients' associations provide information about preparations for power outages and earthquake disasters. For instance, during the Great East Japan Earthquake and subsequent rolling blackouts, patients' associations encouraged patients to contact their service providers via mass media, which helped resolve the concerns of many patients. It is important that various professionals and organizations around patients continue to work in close collaboration to improve disaster preparedness.

References

1. Gas Medicina. 2016,34. K.K. Gas Review.
2. Tohyama K, Kishida R, editors. NPO Japan Respiratory Disorder Patient Information Center Questionnaire survey report about chronic respiratory disease patients. Tokyo: NPO Japan Respiratory Disorder Patient Information Center; 2015. p. 84.
3. Japan Industrial and Medical Gases Association. Guidelines for streamlining the emergency/disaster response systems for the maintenance service providers for home oxygen delivery devices. Tokyo: Japan Industrial and Medical Gases Association; 2017.
4. Kida K, Motegi T, editors. Countermeasures against major disasters for patients with chronic respiratory disease: information for team approach. Tokyo: Medical Review; 2016. p. 212.
5. The Ministry of Health, Labour and Welfare. Project for furthering the approvals of medical devices to promote in-home medical care: an investigative report on the needs for medical devices in in-home medical care.2013.
6. The Japanese Respiratory Society. Guidelines for the diagnosis and treatment of COPD (chronic obstructive pulmonary disease). 4th ed; 2013. p. 103–4.
7. The Japanese Respiratory Society. Guideline for noninvasive positive pressure (NPPV). 2nd ed; 2015. p. 41–7.
8. Company A. (2017). Preparations for disasters.

Chapter 9
Aggravation of the Existing Respiratory Diseases by the Loss or Difficulty in Supplying of Medicines and Medical Application: What Happened and What Measurements Should the Community and the Patient and His Family Do When the Medicines for the Existing Respiratory Disease Are Lost or Not Supplied?

Yuko Komase, Takahiro Tsuburai, and Naoya Hida

Abstract Japan is subject to frequent natural disasters. In patients with respiratory diseases, continuous treatment is needed from the acute phase through the chronic phase of a disaster. When a disaster is divided into the acute, subacute, and chronic phases, medication shortages are expected during the acute phase, which delays the distribution of medications and prevents patients from obtaining enough medications. Given this premise, measures are needed to allow many patients to receive treatment equally during the acute phase. During patient education, medical professionals should encourage patients to stockpile necessary medications to be prepared for the acute phase of a disaster and should provide action plans for patients. During the subacute phase, medication stockpiles start to increase, thereby gradually allowing for the provision of regular treatment to patients. During the chronic phase, many residents tend to live in isolation, and patients need continued support.

Keywords Medication shortages · Acute phase of a disaster · Chronic phase of a disaster · The distribution of medications · Action plans for patients

---

Y. Komase (✉) · T. Tsuburai · N. Hida
Department of Respiratory Internal Medicine, St. Marianna University, School of Medicine, Yokohama-City Seibu Hospital, Yokohama, Kanagawa, Japan
e-mail: yukomase@marianna-u.ac.jp

K. Fujimoto (ed.), *Disaster and Respiratory Diseases*,
Respiratory Disease Series: Diagnostic Tools and Disease Managements,
https://doi.org/10.1007/978-981-13-2598-4_9

9.1 Introduction

Japan is subject to frequent natural disasters. Large earthquakes have struck the country roughly once every 10 years. One of the most memorable ones is the Great Hanshin-Awaji Earthquake of 1995. Since then, the country has been hit by multiple large earthquakes in succession. According to the World Risk Report 2017, Japan has, by far, the highest chance among the developed countries of getting affected by natural disasters (39.6%), followed by the United States (12.0%) and the United Kingdom (11.6%) (Fig. 9.1) [1]. Among the various natural disasters, earthquakes are the most frequent in Japan. In fact, 10% of earthquakes with a magnitude of 5.0 and above and more than 20% of those with a magnitude of 6.0 and above worldwide have occurred in and around Japan [2].

Data presented by the Cabinet Office showed a worldwide increase in intense floods and localized heavy rainfalls with rising temperatures. Given this trend, the role that medical care should fulfill for patients with chronic diseases, who are vulnerable to disasters, is becoming increasingly important [3].

Regarding earthquakes, the Great Hanshin-Awaji Earthquake struck major cities, and rescue operations and medical activities were carried out mostly during the acute phase. In contrast, the Great East Japan Earthquake affected many elderly residents over a considerably large area, thereby necessitating long-term medical assistance. These experiences revealed that the "medical care" needed can differ in quality and quantity depending on the size and location of the affected region [4, 5].

Besides earthquakes, Japan also experiences other natural disasters each year, including typhoons, floods, landslides, and volcanic eruptions.

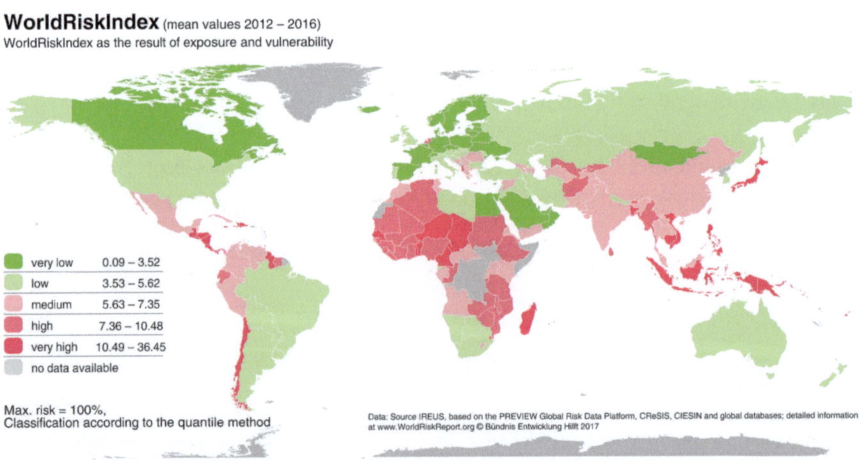

Fig. 9.1 The WorldRiskIndex states the risk of an extreme natural event leading to a disaster in 171 countries. Japan has the highest chance among the developed countries of getting affected by natural disasters

The age distribution in Japan shows a rapid progression in population aging, and increasing emphasis has been placed on the importance of caring for elderly patients with chronic diseases—some of whom may even have multiple diseases—in times of disasters.

In terms of respiratory diseases, measures are needed not only for patients with acute conditions caused by the disaster but also for those with chronic respiratory diseases, such as asthma or chronic obstructive pulmonary disease (COPD), because many of these patients will need continued treatment. Moreover, chronic respiratory diseases are likely to exacerbate after a disaster. Inhaled medications play a vital role in the treatment of respiratory diseases. However, unlike oral medications, they come in a variety of forms and are therefore not suitable for stockpiling. Additionally, an inhaled medication cannot readily be substituted by another medication because of differences in inhalation devices. In many cases, a pharmaceutical association's list of stockpile medications contains many oral medications for chronic respiratory diseases, but only a few inhaled medications [5, 6].

This paper discusses how medical professionals should respond to future disasters and associated issues, as well as the steps patients can take to be prepared for such disasters.

9.2 The State of Chronic Diseases in Times of Natural Disasters

Some of the potential influences that a disaster may have over patients with chronic disease are (1) the cessation of medication delivery due to the collapse of the medical care system; (2) the spread of infectious diseases, exposure to cold, and aggravation of the disease because of air pollution and other factors; and (3) mental stress caused by the disaster. In the Great East Japan Earthquake, asthma exacerbations were reported in Fukushima prefecture because of a cessation of the provision of anti-asthmatic medications. Even among patients who could continue taking anti-asthmatic medications, a significantly higher incidence of asthma exacerbations was reported among those who had severe anxiety over the disaster [7, 8]. A report indicated that the conditions of patients with COPD were exacerbated because of the lack of treatment medications during the subacute phase [9, 10]. The incidence of tsunami lung was also noted along with the onset or aggravation of interstitial pneumonia associated with the inhalation of fine dust during post-disaster debris removal, home repairs, etc. [11].

As described so far, patients with chronic respiratory diseases often experience a deterioration of their conditions because of a disaster. For patients who are most vulnerable to disasters, it is extremely important to continue receiving appropriate treatment as much as possible for their prognoses as well. Having a medication supply during the acute phase (within 3 days after a disaster) [12] and subacute phase (from 4 days to 3 weeks after a disaster) can affect treatment continuation in patients. The chronic phase (from 3 weeks to 5 years after a disaster) is a time to restore the regional medical care system. However, this is also a time when the patients' mental stress is further intensified; residents may withdraw and sometimes die alone in temporary housing. Therefore, it is necessary to restore the medical care system and take appropriate measures for patients with chronic diseases [9].

9.3 Medication Delivery System

The impact of a natural disaster varies according to the size of the disaster and situation of the affected region. In foreign countries, the availability of medications differs between an urban area with relatively many pharmacies and a large region with a few pharmacies. When considering the provision of medications, we should separate the acute phase from the subacute phase, during which medications become more available [13].

1. Preparing medications for the acute phase: Saving human lives is the number one priority in the super-acute phase, but this is also the time when chronic respiratory diseases tend to deteriorate. It is desirable that patients themselves prepare about a week's extra supply of medications, along with their prescription records, to bring with them when being evacuated. However, this may not be possible for some patients. Therefore, each region has its own designated places to stockpile basic medications in preparation for disasters. Pharmaceutical associations have created disaster countermeasure manuals, including a list of the most basic medications needed [6].
2. Preparing medications for the subacute phase: Medical professionals like us have little to no knowledge about the distribution of medicinal products. In the Great East Japan Earthquake, employees of pharmaceutical wholesalers had previously collected information on the demand for medicinal products in local areas through their routine product delivery and price negotiation, which helped secure nearly enough medications to meet the demand a few days after the disaster. Damaged equipment and inventory shortages could be overcome through cooperation that went beyond the framework of corporations. This experience has shown the possibility that wholesalers' distribution channels may be the most useful in the delivery of medications in the event of a major natural disaster in the future. At the prefectural level, efforts have been underway to establish a collaboration system for the delivery of medicinal products during a disaster. The Federation of Japan Pharmaceutical Wholesalers Association has also reported challenges in the delivery of medicinal products during a natural disaster [12].
3. Current issues

   - On the basis of the lessons learned from the Great East Japan Earthquake, more specific measures need to be developed, including how to streamline the delivery of medicinal products from pharmaceutical wholesalers to first-aid stations and evacuation shelters.

- In connection with the delivery of medicinal products from pharmaceutical manufacturers to pharmaceutical wholesalers, manufacturing or logistic hubs are too concentrated. Therefore, risk distribution and alternative measures are needed.
- Measures for the delivery of medicinal products need to involve supply chains, and collaboration with the government or multiple municipalities is essential in times of large-scale disasters. In the future, it will be necessary to develop a system of comprehensive disaster countermeasures that go beyond the framework of individual industries and municipalities.

In the Great East Japan Earthquake, the system for the delivery of medicinal products to medical institutes/pharmacies was restored within 3 days of the disaster, but the provision of medications at evacuation shelters was delayed because of the delay in sorting out the large amounts of medications brought in. There were also left-over medications, indicating the need for the establishment of a more organized, well-balanced medication delivery system to improve the situation.

As a future countermeasure for earthquakes and other disasters, the use of a regular wholesale distribution system would be most suitable considering the current circumstances in Japan. Moreover, the volume of medication delivery from pharmaceutical manufacturers to pharmaceutical wholesalers needs to be examined.

9.4 Characteristics of Each Type of Respiratory Disease

Here we focus on bronchial asthma, COPD, interstitial lung diseases, and lung cancer as typical respiratory diseases. At the beginning of a disaster, however, the incidence of infectious diseases increases. In particular, the Great East Japan Earthquake occurred during the winter season and respiratory infections such as pneumonia were noted early on [14–16]. Inhaled medications are the basic medication for the treatment of respiratory diseases; however, their drawback is that they come in a variety of inhalation devices. Therefore, it is difficult to stockpile all types of inhaled medications for disasters, and patients may possibly be given a medication that they have never used before, thereby causing the discontinuation of their treatment. Unlike tablets, which can be distributed to patients from a minimum of one tablet per person, stockpiling a sufficient number of inhalation devices to distribute one per patient is expected to be difficult.

9.4.1 Bronchial Asthma

Bronchial asthma is a condition that can be worsened by stress. Patients with no prior experience of having an asthma attack may experience one for the first time during a disaster. At the time of the Kumamoto earthquakes, there were patients who had their first asthma attack, which was difficult to distinguish from common cold. To diagnose these patients in a situation without proper testing equipment, Yoshimura et al. reported that having patients inhale short-acting β2-agonists (SABAs) helped determine the condition to some extent (personal communication). To allow many patients to inhale SABAs, paper cups were used in lieu of spacers, and these were found to be useful.

For patients who have previously been diagnosed with asthma, it is necessary to keep it under control by using inhaled corticosteroids (ICSs) and other medications during a stable period. However, many patients do not use their ICSs regularly as they should, and some of them are likely to experience an asthma exacerbation triggered by a natural disaster. Treatment should be initiated quickly in these patients as well.

Some of the medications commonly used in patients with asthma during a stable period are ICSs, ICSs/long-acting β2-agonists (LABAs), and long-acting muscarinic antagonists (LAMAs). For the super-acute phase, it is necessary to prepare at least ICSs (currently, ICS/LABA has the highest rate of use in Japan, and thus, stockpiling ICS/LABA is considered practical), along with SABAs for patients having an asthma attack. Although there are a variety of inhalation devices, it is desirable to stockpile the inhaled medications that are used most commonly in the region and are easy to use. However, as mentioned before, stockpiling ICSs is quite difficult compared to stockpiling oral medications, which can be distributed flexibly according to the number of doses needed by each patient, because each patient needs one inhalation device. One solution for this is to prepare medications that can be used with a paper-cup spacer to allow many patients to use it. As for patients with severe asthma, some may take oral steroids regularly and others may use antibodies. Antibodies are usually used once a month to every 2 weeks and are thus not needed right away in times of disasters. However, some of the patients who were regularly taking corticosteroids may have developed adrenal insufficiency. Therefore, it is absolutely necessary to stockpile corticosteroids as an emergency medication in case of further aggravation of their conditions.

It is also important to give consideration to patients with aspirin-induced asthma (i.e., with nonsteroidal anti-inflammatory drug intolerance), which is a type of severe asthma. The problem of additives should also be considered. When ICS or ICS/LABA is needed, the number of inhalation devices obtainable and their storage space may be limited. One way to resolve this problem is to administer medications via a pressurized metered-dose inhaler with a paper cup used as a spacer. As analgesics, either acetaminophen (less than 300 mg per dose) or a selective COX-2 inhibitor (celecoxib) is needed. An asthma exacerbation is often triggered by an infectious disease, which is usually viral but can sometimes be bacterial. Therefore, it is important to provide antimicrobial agents that are effective against respiratory infections.

9.4.2 COPD

Bronchodilators are the mainstay in the treatment of COPD. Unlike bronchial asthma, a cessation of the inhaled medication does not immediately lead to the worsening of COPD, but can still be a trigger for an acute exacerbation. LAMA inhalers are the desired medication for stockpiling; however, as COPD is a common illness in the elderly, preparing β2-agonist patches is also a good idea. Many medications used in patients with bronchial asthma are also used to treat COPD. The most important medications to prepare are the ones used to treat acute exacerbations: antimicrobials and oral corticosteroids. According to the guidelines published by the Japanese Association for Infectious Diseases, respiratory quinolones should actively be considered as antimicrobials to treat elderly patients, patients with COPD, and patients with obsolete pulmonary tuberculosis [17]. SABAs are used for the relief of asthma attacks, but they also demonstrate high effectiveness in alleviating breathing difficulty in COPD and should thus be used actively in patients with COPD who are prone to breathing problems.

9.4.3 Interstitial Pneumonia

Interstitial pneumonia may be induced by exposure to fine dust emitted from post-disaster debris removal or home repairs during the chronic phase. Interstitial pneumonia that developed prior to a disaster may also become exacerbated [11]. In particular, the mainstays in the treatment of idiopathic pulmonary fibrosis are anti-fibrotic agents, which are used to prevent a decline in the pulmonary function and acute exacerbations. However, as anti-fibrotic agents do not bring about rapid changes in the condition, they do not need to be included in the medication stockpile for the super-acute phase. Interstitial pneumonia can be acutely exacerbated by infections and other factors, and thus requires treatment with corticosteroids. However, treatment delays can often lead to serious outcomes. Therefore, if a patient experiences an exacerbation of interstitial pneumonia, the patient should immediately be transferred to an area where sufficient medical care is available.

Additionally, in patients with interstitial pneumonia who have been undergoing steroid treatment, a cessation of treatment can increase the risk for an acute exacerbation. Hence, continued treatment is important for these patients.

9.4.4 Lung Cancer

Lung cancer may be detected at an advanced stage because of a delay in seeking medical care. Additionally, in patients undergoing chemotherapy, running out of the medications may lead to a rapid progression of the cancer. Since it is difficult to include anticancer agents in emergency medications, patients should be transferred to an area where sufficient medical care is available.

9.4.5 Mycobacterial Infections

The prevalence of mycobacterial infections among elderly people has become problematic in recent years. In particular, being forced to live in unfamiliar environments in times of disasters may cause a decline in the immune system, resulting in the onset of tuberculosis. Patients undergoing anti-tuberculosis treatment need to continue their treatment, but if any change occurs in the condition, it is desirable that they receive medical care outside the disaster-struck region. Nontuberculous mycobacterial infections have become more prevalent than tuberculosis in recent years, and they are highly likely to lead to bronchiectasis as a secondary infection, as well as to the aggravation of the mycobacterial infection itself. This can be addressed using medications that are effective against common respiratory infections.

9.5 Regional Countermeasures and Their Challenges

9.5.1 Disaster Countermeasures Taken by Medical Professionals

On the basis of various experiences gained in the past, many disaster response systems have been established across Japan.

9.5.1.1 Regional Situations

Yokohama Pharmaceutical Association has selected about 100 pharmacies as rolling stock pharmacies to be prepared for natural disasters. Each of these pharmacies stores medications for 80 to 100 patients, and these medications are managed by pharmacists at all times. This system allows for the provision of medications during the super-acute phase of a disaster [18].

Miyagi, Wakayama, Hiroshima, Tottori, and Oita prefectures have launched mobile pharmacies to realize the delivery of medications to remote areas by vehicles [19]. Thus, regional medication delivery systems vary based on their situations, and each region aims to establish a system that works best for it.

Manuals cannot be followed exactly as they are, because the support needed can be different depending on the scale of the disaster, time of year (season), place, time of day, and other factors. With the advancement in information-communication technologies, people have more information.

With the advancement in information-communication technologies, manuals should be modified according to the situation. Therefore, it is necessary to act in a creative and flexible manner according to individual circumstances.

9.5.1.2 Disaster Countermeasure Manual Developed by the Japan Pharmaceutical Association (JPA)

Pharmaceutical departments of hospitals and pharmacies need to collaborate with local pharmaceutical associations and hospitals in selecting and creating the lists of medications for stockpiling, confirming medication delivery routes with wholesalers, providing patient education (to teach patients about their medications, means of communication in case of an emergency, etc.), grasping which patients will require assistance, etc. Furthermore, the JPA has expanded support resources from local to prefectural pharmaceutical associations and shows in its manual the measures to be implemented by nearby prefectures [6]. However, the JPA's list of anti-asthmatic and COPD medications to be carried during the subacute phase includes only Theo-Dur®, Sultanol® Inhaler®, Venetlin® for inhalation, Hokunalin® Tape, and Neophyllin® injection and does not contain most of the inhaled medications usually used for asthma and COPD during a stable period. It is necessary to contrive a way to provide inhaled medications for many patients safely by using minimum space.

9.5.2 Patient Education

In addition to the training of medical professionals, educating patients to promote their understanding is an important part of preparing for an emergency. In doing so, medical professionals need to ensure that patients fully understand their diseases and know what to do in case of an acute exacerbation. In actual clinical settings, many patients request for the prescription of about a week's extra supply of medications out of concern for running out of them. Medical professionals need to make sure that patients understand the diagnosis and severity of their diseases and names of the medications they are currently taking, as many of them do not. Since patients are not properly informed of the severity of their asthma/COPD by their doctors, most of them are not aware of how serious their condition is, despite the fact that they regularly take oral corticosteroids. At the very least, patients should be informed of the diagnosis and severity of their condition. As the names of medications can be complicated, and are often in katakana, they are difficult for Japanese patients to memorize. Medical professionals should repeatedly inform their patients of the names and roles of their medications, whether these medications can be discontinued if pressed by circumstances, how many days they can go without taking them, etc.

9.5.3 Development of Action Plans

What to do at the time of an exacerbation: It is important to provide patients with an action plan, usually in written form, and regularly check their level of understanding (a written action plan). An action plan defines an exacerbation and describes what to do if the condition is exacerbated. An action plan for patients with bronchial asthma describes asthma attacks and their severity levels, along with appropriate treatments for each severity, such as appropriate dose increases in ICSs, how to use other types of bronchodilators, the timing to take oral corticosteroids, and the timing to seek medical attention. For patients with COPD, some facilities provide education on the symptoms indicative of an infection and the use of antimicrobial agents. However, since many patients with COPD are elderly, most facilities recommend seeking medical attention, rather than taking emergency medications. In comparison, disaster-specific action plans should also include the types and doses of the medications regularly taken, list of medications for exacerbations and how to use them, and what to do in case of a medication shortage. Regarding patients with COPD, the possibility of a shortage of oxygen should be considered for those receiving home oxygen therapy; it is desirable that their action plans include how to adjust the level of oxygen. In many cases, it takes roughly a week before a certain level of medication delivery can resume, but whether sufficient amounts of medications, especially inhaled medications, are available then is uncertain. Patients are usually encouraged to stock about a week's worth of medications, but they should also be informed of what to do when they are running out of their medications. In the future, it is necessary to have patients carry a patient card containing details on their treatment, including their asthma severity and contraindicated medications, and ensure that patients fully understand their conditions before a disaster occurs. Many regional pharmaceutical associations utilize patients' prescription records, and an increasing number of patients are bringing their prescription records with them when visiting a hospital. It is desirable to integrate a written action plan into a prescription record in some form.

9.5.4 Patient Support in Times of Disasters

Emergency medications delivered during the subacute phase of a disaster may not be exactly the same as the medications patients have been using. Even with the same indications, some emergency medications are likely to be somewhat different from the ones patients are accustomed to. In that case, medical professionals must be fully aware that the potency of inhaled medications varies according to the device. In particular, patients using inhaled medications may be given a medication they may have never inhaled before because of the difference in the inhalation device. In such a situation, special attention should be paid by doctors, pharmacists, nurses, and other medical professionals to check if the patients are able to inhale the medication. Although medical professionals are busy during the subacute phase because of limited medical resources, they need to not only hand out inhaled medications to patients but also make sure that the patients can use them properly. This does not need to be done by doctors. Rather, it would be more efficient to get assistance from many other medical staff members. In the unfamiliar environment of an evacuation shelter, patients may miss the timing to take the medication or fail to use the medication properly for fear of bothering other people around them. In particular, elderly patients may have trouble with inhalation techniques and fail to inhale the medication because of their unfamiliarity with the device. Therefore, medical professionals must thoroughly check on how patients are using the inhalation device; if they still cannot use it properly, the use of oral corticosteroids may need to be considered as an emergency measure.

9.5.5 Streamlining the Environment

Patients with asthma or COPD do not look obviously different to other people. Therefore, when these patients take preventive measures against exacerbations, other people affected by the disaster may find their situation difficult to understand. For example, using clean bedding to prevent an asthma attack or not participating in post-disaster debris cleanup to avoid inhaling fine dust may not be understood by other residents, as they are under extreme stress. To be prepared for such situations, the Japanese Society of Pediatric Allergy and Clinical Immunology has created a pamphlet (Fig. 9.2) [20, 21]. However, no such information materials have yet been created for adult patients. In this aspect, efforts should be made to develop pamphlets for adult patients, in the same format throughout Japan if possible, along with posters that allow medical professionals to promote an understanding about patients with asthma/COPD among other people affected by a disaster.

9.5.6 What Type of Patients Should Be Moved to the Area Where Sufficient Medical Care Is Available?

Owing to a disruption in the medical care system, it is difficult to provide continuous treatment for patients with severe respiratory disease at evacuation shelters. With regard to patients with severe respiratory insufficiency, asthma attacks that do not improve after standard treatment, severe pneumonia, acute exacerbations of

Dealing with allergies during a disaster

Dealing with asthma in children

Living in an unfamiliar environment can result in a high rate of asthma attacks. To prevent such exacerbations, please remember the following points and consult with the staff at evacuation shelters or the local government when encountering a problem:

Avoid objects that trigger an asthma attack (causes).

- **Dust mites (can be found in bedding and dust), animals (such as dogs and cats), smoke (such as cigarettes, open fire, and mosquito coils), fine dust emitted from post-disaster debris, etc.**

  (Preventive measures)
  - Apply a mask or clean towel over your mouth to avoid inhaling them.
  - Stay away from such places or move yourself to some other place.

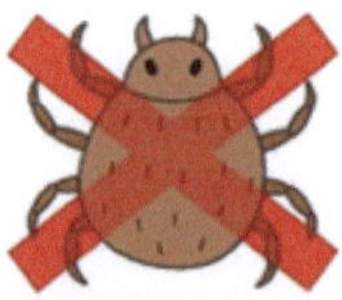

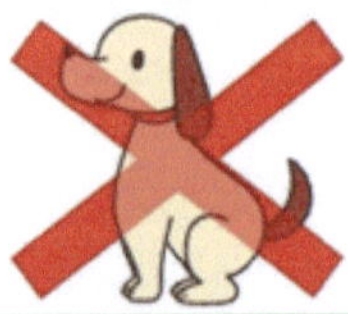

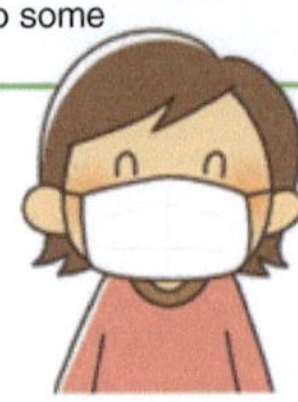

Continue taking preventive medications for asthma attacks every day. Consult with a doctor in the following cases:

- **If you are out of your preventive medications or running low on them**
- **If you still have coughing fits or asthma attacks repeatedly despite continuing your preventive medications**
- **Even though you have a nebulizer,**
  - **(1) You are not allowed to use an emergency electric power source. (Consult with a doctor so that you can be given priority for using it.)**
  - **(2) You do not have an electric power source. (By switching to an aerosol inhaler with a supplemental device called a spacer, you will no longer need an electric power source. If you cannot obtain a spacer, you can substitute it with a paper cup with a small hole punched at the bottom.)**

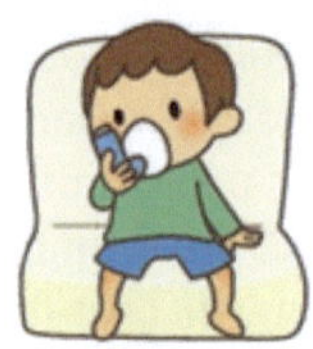

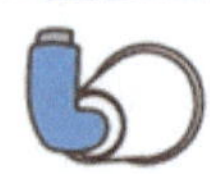

If an asthma attack occurs,

- **Give the patient water and tell the patient to take slow and deep breaths. Administer the asthma relief medication (oral or inhalable) and have the patient lean back and rest. If the patient still wakes up repeatedly because of discomfort or suddenly sits down because of shortness of breath, the patient needs to be examined by a doctor.**

Consultation services on allergies in children in a time of a disaster (free of charge)
▶ E-mail consultation: sup_jasp@jspaci.jp

Japanese Society of Pediatric Allergy and Clinical Immunology
Website URL: http://www.jspaci.jp/

Fig. 9.2 The Japanese Society of Pediatric Allergy and Clinical Immunology has created a pamphlet to prevent an asthma attack

COPD, and acute exacerbations of interstitial pulmonary diseases, and those undergoing lung cancer treatment, it is necessary to consider transferring them to an area where sufficient medical care is available as soon as possible.

9.6 Conclusion

To cope with the shortage of drugs in the event of a disaster, preparations should be made before the disaster occurs. The patient needs to prepare the medicine according to the action plan as an emergency response. Although only minimal amounts of drugs must be stocked for use during the acute phase of a disaster, stockpiling of inhaled medicines, which are especially important for respiratory diseases, should be enhanced. In addition, minimal amounts of drugs such as steroids and antibacterial drugs are necessary for patients with acute exacerbation, but transporting these patients to hospitals with proper equipment as soon as possible is an important consideration.

References

1. Kirch L, Luther S, Mucke P et al. WorldRiskReport- Analysis and prospects 2017. Bündnis Entwicklung Hilft. 2017. https://reliefweb.int/report/world/world-risk-report-2017. Accessed 6 Feb 2018
2. Japan Institute of Country-ology and Engineering. http://www.jice.or.jp/knowledge/japan/commentary12#jump_01. Accessed 6 Feb 2018 (in Japanese)
3. Early Warning Sub-Committee of the Inter-Ministerial Committee on International Cooperation for Disaster Reduction Government of Japan. Japan's Natural Disaster Early Warning Systems and International Cooperative Efforts. Cabinet Office, Government of Japan. 2006. http://bousaigojp/kokusai/kyoryoku Accessed 6 Feb 2018 (in Japanese)
4. Nagamatsu S, Maekawa T, Ujike Y, et al. The earthquake and tsunami—observations by Japanese physicians since the11 March catastrophe. Crit Care. 2011;15:167.
5. Otani Y, Ando T, Atobe K, et al. Comparison of two larger earthquakes: the 2008 Sichuan Earthquake and the 2011 East Japan Earthquake. Keio J Med. 2012;61:35–9.
6. Japan Pharmaceutical Association. 2015. http://www.nichiyaku.or.jp/saigai2016/files/sr20160415.pdf#search=%27%E7%81%BD%E5%AE%B3%E3%80%81%E8%96%AC%E5%89%A4%E5%82%99%E8%93%84%27. Accessed 6 Feb 2018 (in Japanese)
7. Fukuhara A, Sato S, Uematsu M, et al. Impact of the 3.11 Disaster in Fukushima on Asthma Control. Am J Respir Crit Care Med. 2012;186:1309–10.
8. Kobayashi S, Hanagama M, Yamanda S, Satoh H, Tokuda S, Kobayashi M, Ueda S, Suzuki S, Yanai M. The impact of a large-scale natural disaster on patients with chronic obstructive pulmonary disease: the aftermath of the 2011 Great East Japan Earthquake. Respir Investig. 2013;51:17–23.
9. Yamanouchi K. Medical disease learned from the Great East Japan Earthquake-Feature, Treatment and Prevention; 2 Respiratory Diseases. Nippon Naika Gakkai Zasshi. 2014;103:551–6. in Japanese

10. Ohkochi S, Shibuya R, Yanai M, Nukiwa T. Deterioration in regional health status after the acute phase of a great disaster: respiratory physicians' experiences of the Great East Japan Earthquake. Respir Investig. 2013;51:50–5.
11. Ohkouchi S, et al. Fatal acute interstitial pneumonia a worker making chips from wooden debris generated by the Great East Japan earthquake and tsunami. Respir Investig. 2012;50(4):129.
12. Japan Pharmaceutical Wholesalers Association. 2015. www.jpwa.or.jp/jpwa/pdf/topics_201601_01.pdf. Accessed 6 Feb 2018 (in Japanese)
13. Fuse A, Shuto Y, Ando F, et al. Medical relief activities conducted by Nippon Medical School in the acute phase of the Great East Japan Earthquake 2011. J Nihon Med Sch. 2011;78:397–400.
14. Suzuki M, Uwano C, Ohrui T, et al. Shelter-acquired pneumonia after a catastrophic earthquake in Japan. J Am Geriatr Soc. 2011;59:1968–70.
15. Koudio IK, Alunid S, Kamigaki T, et al. Infectious diseases following natural disasters: prevention and control measures. Expert Rev Anti-Infect Ther. 2012;10:95–104.
16. Aghababian RV, Teuacher J. Infectious diseases following major disasters. Ann Emergency Med. 1992;21:362–7.
17. Mikasa K, Aoki N, Aoki Y, et al. Infectious Diseases: The Japanese Association for Infectious Diseases/Japanese Society of Chemotherapy—The JAID/JSC Guide to Clinical Management of Infectious Disease/Guideline-preparing Committee Respiratory Infectious Disease WG. J Infect Chemotherapy. 2016;22:S1–S65.
18. Yokohama Pharmaceutical Association. http://www.hamayaku.or.jp/saigai-2016-5.html. Accessed 6 Feb 2018 (in Japanese)
19. Oita Pharmaceutical Association. http://www.oitakenyaku.or.jp/manage/wp-content/uploads/2014/09/Mobile-Pharmacy.pdf. Accessed 6 Feb 2018 (in Japanese)
20. Adachi Y, Fujiwara T. Dealing with asthma/allergy ailments in children during a disaster: a report on the Great East Japan Earthquake and proposals for future actions—5. Countermeasure pamphlet (2) Asthma. Jpn J Pediatr Allergy Clin Immunol. 2011;25:742–5.
21. Matsui T. Dealing with asthma/allergy ailments in children during a disaster: a report on the Great East Japan Earthquake and proposals for future actions—4. Local assistance. Jpn J Pediatr Allergy Clin Immunol. 2011;25:734–8.

Chapter 10
Aggravation of the Existing Respiratory Diseases due to Transportation Stoppage, Closure of the Medical Institution, and Shortage of Doctors: What Measurements Securing Health Resources and What Actions for the Supply of Health Resources Are Talked About?

Masaru Yanai

Abstract Large-scale natural disasters affect large geographic areas significantly impacting people, infrastructure, public health, and medical regimens. Such catastrophic occurrences can result in the aggravation of preexisting chronic diseases as well as the development of acute diseases such as infectious or cardiovascular diseases. In order to effectively utilize the limited medical resources for the treatment of excessive numbers of casualties during the aftermath of the disaster, it is essential to integrate medical relief updates through a unified chain of command. Healthcare professionals should educate patients with chronic respiratory diseases so that they can personally manage their own diseases. Healthcare professionals should also educate patients about general disaster preparedness. In order to continue medication for chronic respiratory diseases and/or long-term oxygen therapy (LTOT) during the aftermath of a disaster, accessible measures such as mobile dispensing pharmacies or LTOT centers might be considered.

Keywords Tohoku Earthquake · Ishinomaki Zone Joint Relief Team · Self-management Risk management cycle

---

M. Yanai
Department of Respiratory Medicine, Japanese Red Cross Ishinomaki Hospital, Ishinomaki, Miyagi, Japan

K. Fujimoto (ed.), *Disaster and Respiratory Diseases*,
Respiratory Disease Series: Diagnostic Tools and Disease Managements,
https://doi.org/10.1007/978-981-13-2598-4_10

10.1 Introduction

Large-scale natural disasters affect large geographic areas significantly impacting the population and environment. Such catastrophic occurrences can result in extraordinary levels of human casualties and disruption of infrastructure, environment, economy, national morale, and government functions [1]. Medical facilities and emergency response organizations are some of the many community-built structures that experience such physical devastation. Local medical staff are unable to assume their normal roles due to losses in personnel and facilities. Roads and railway lines often become unpassable, oftentimes resulting in failure to transport medical relief supplies and emergency medical teams.

Preexisting chronic respiratory diseases can be aggravated both during and in the aftermath of a disaster, due to a variety of factors including discontinuation of usual medical treatments, an austere disaster environment, and severely damaged public health.

In this chapter, I will report what Japanese Red Cross Ishinomaki Hospital staff experienced and what we learned during the aftermath of the 2011 Tohoku Earthquake in Ishinomaki Medical Zone, Miyagi, Japan—one of the most severely affected areas by the earthquake and tsunami.

10.2 Disaster Situation of Ishinomaki Medical Zone by Tohoku Earthquake

10.2.1 Damage Status of Ishinomaki Medical Zone by Tohoku Earthquake

The 2011 Tohoku Earthquake and tsunami destroyed vast areas of Japan's eastern seaboard. The Ishinomaki Medical Zone, which consists of Ishinomaki city, Higashi-Matsushima city, and Onagawa town, is located on the northeast Pacific coast of Honshu Island. Before the earthquake, the population of the Ishinomaki Medical Zone was 220,000 people covering 72,000 km^2. Residential areas, commercial and industrial areas, municipal and public offices, schools, and hospitals were distributed along the coastline. The Ishinomaki Medical Zone suffered the largest number of civilian casualties in Japan; nearly 6000 people, 30% of total civilian casualties directly related to the earthquake and tsunami, were killed or are still missing. 90% of these victims drowned, and approximately half of them were over 70 years old.

16% of the area was inundated up to 18.5 m, and 60% of houses were totally or severely destroyed. There were ten hospitals in the medical zone; two were completely destroyed, six were inundated and temporarily ceased their medical operations, and one lost functionality due to power failure, water outage, and building damage. Only one hospital, Japanese Red Cross (JRC) Ishinomaki Hospital, a regional disaster base hospital with 402 beds, escaped the tsunami and perfectly preserved its hospital function due to the hospital's seismic isolation structure, backup generation, and water storage.

Out of 78 clinics in the medical zone, 10 were totally destroyed, 17 were severely damaged, 23 were moderately damaged, and the remaining 28 clinics were either slightly damaged or untouched.

Out of 97 dispensing pharmacies, 38 were completely destroyed, and 31 were severely damaged. Even slightly damaged or relatively untouched, medical facilities failed to work because of area-wide power and water supply failure.

10.2.2 Damages to Infrastructure in Ishinomaki Medical Zone

The Tohoku Earthquake and the accompanying tsunami destroyed most of the medical and healthcare facilities as described above. The municipal government building was also severely inundated. Roads along such inundated areas were completely blocked by heaps of wreckage and masses of sludge as thick as several decimeters over the ground and wreckage. Other roads including expressways and trunk roads were also partially destroyed and obstructed. Water and sewer service, gas supply, and electricity were totally unavailable in the medical zone. Telecommunication services, except for satellite phone service, were inaccessible in most of the area.

Maximum outage of electricity, water, and gas in the medical zone was 194, 123, and 64 days, respectively.

The JR East Senseki-Line, the line between Sendai and Ishinomaki, was discontinued. It took 50 months for it to be completely restored.

10.3 Disaster Medicine at Japanese Red Cross Ishinomaki Hospital

10.3.1 Disaster Medicine of the Acute and Subacute Phase

Nearly 4000 emergency patients visited JRC Ishinomaki Hospital within the week immediately following the disaster. This is in stark contrast to the more usual burden of 60 emergency patients per day—a tenfold increase in emergency visits.

All scheduled hospitalizations were canceled, and emergency admissions were accepted only during the first 60 days following the earthquake. The 1769 patients that were admitted to the hospital during this period included 322 patients with respiratory diseases accounting for 18.2% of the total admissions. This percentage was significantly higher than those of corresponding periods over the past 2 years (10.2% in 2010 and 11.6% in 2009) [2].

While the total number of admissions peaked within the first 10 days, the number of admissions for patients diagnosed with respiratory diseases continued to increase for 20 more days [2].

We compared the disease distribution between 2011 and the previous 2 years. The JRC Ishinomaki Hospital is the only respiratory center in the medical region, and most respiratory patients in the region were hospitalized here even before the disaster. There were four times more pneumonia (the most common of these respiratory diseases) cases in 2011 compared with the 2 previous years. Similar increases were seen in admissions from COPD exacerbations and asthma attacks. Admissions for symptoms of lung cancer or other respiratory diseases did not increase significantly within this period [2].

10.3.2 Wide-Area Evacuation of Patients from Japanese Red Cross Ishinomaki Hospital

In JRC Ishinomaki Hospital, 1769 patients were urgently hospitalized for the first 60 days after the earthquake, twice as many as in either of the preceding 2 years. Three hundred twenty-two patients were admitted with respiratory diseases—three times more than in past years.

In order to continue accepting newly admitted emergency patients, we had to transfer a number of patients out of the hospital. Every morning, we selected patients who had become stable enough to endure transportation and who seemed to need long hospitalization, and then we asked them to accept wide-area transportation outside the stricken zone. Responsible doctors from the emergency department and staff from the regional medical liaison office worked together to decide appropriate hospital and transportation measures. During the 60 days after the earthquake, 534 patients were transported to hospitals or healthcare facilities outside the severely stricken area; 180 of them were respiratory patients.

10.3.3 Long-Term Oxygen Therapy (LTOT) Patients

There were 250 patients who had received LTOT in the Ishinomaki Medical Zone before the Tohoku Earthquake. Thirty-three of these patients (13%) were killed during the earthquake and tsunami, five times greater than the proportion of deaths when considering the entire population of the area. Eighty-eight LTOT patients who lost electricity or their entire homes voluntarily came to the JRC Ishinomaki Hospital to get oxygen. Between the third and the tenth days following the earthquake, more than 60 patients stayed in the hospital as outpatients. We did not have enough beds in the hospital to accept the enormous number of affected patients. To deal with this problem, we established an LTOT center in the rehabilitation center with 30 oxygen concentrators and 30 cot beds [3]. By vigorous transportation to relatives or hospitals outside the severely affected area, the LTOT center was closed 15 days after the earthquake. During these 15 days, 20% of these LTOT patients suffered from exacerbations of chronic respiratory failure which needed hospitalization, presumably due to interruption of oxygen inhalation and/or medication, getting severely drenched under such cold temperatures, or the crowded conditions in the LTOT center [3].

10.4 Ishinomaki Zone Joint Relief Team

10.4.1 Emergency Shelters in Ishinomaki Medical Zone

It took a week for the water to recede from the inundated area. The Japan Self-Defense Forces (JSDF) rescued many people who had drifted away as a result of the tsunami or had escaped to the upper floors or roofs of submerged buildings. As soon as the water receded, the JSDF removed debris and sludge, which allowed vehicles to travel the roads ensuring smooth transportation of supplies to the affected areas [4].

There were about 300 emergency shelters in the medical zone (Fig. 10.1). As affected people evacuated to the nearest designated location, most shelters were set up in buildings within the inundated areas. The municipal government made a list of emergency shelters with the name of shelters and the number of total evacuees. The

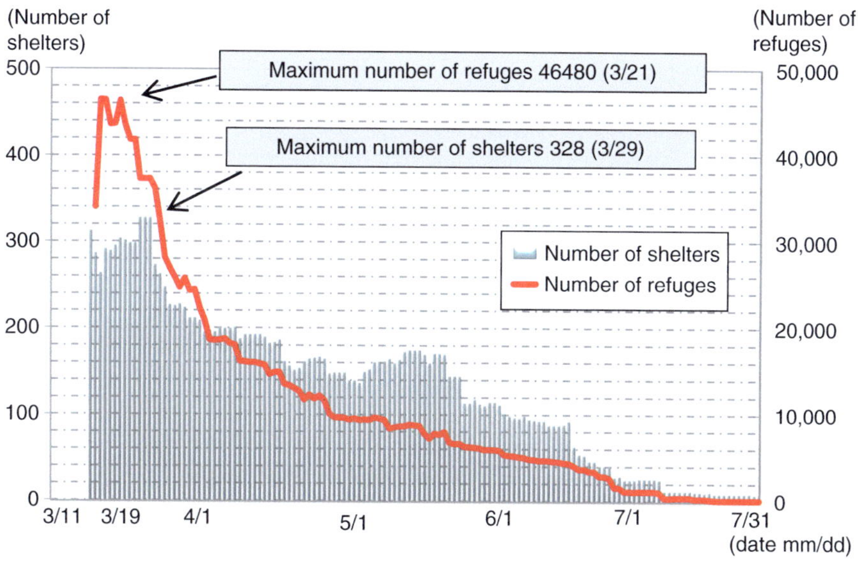

Fig. 10.1 Number of shelters and refugees in the Ishinomaki Medical Zone over time after the Tohoku Earthquake. The number of shelters kept increasing for 3 weeks after the Tohoku Earthquake reaching a maximum of 328 shelters before gradually decreasing to less than 10 shelters by the third month following the earthquake. The number of refugees reached a maximum of 46,480 people, accounting for nearly one-quarter of all local residents

list unfortunately did not provide details about the conditions of the shelters, such as the status of infrastructure stability within evacuation center buildings, or the number of infants, pregnant women, or persons who were disabled or required nursing care.

10.4.2 Establishment of Ishinomaki Zone Joint Relief Team [5]

Within 12 h of the earthquake, medical relief teams began to gather at JRC Ishinomaki Hospital, the designated disaster hospital and the only fully functional hospital in the medical zone. Because detailed and comprehensive disaster information was not initially available, the medical relief teams individually visited both nearby shelters and those in isolated areas according to their own judgment or by the request of the JSDF or the local fire brigades. Their activities were often inefficient; while several teams would spend an entire day at one shelter, other shelters were left without the medical help that they urgently needed.

One week after the earthquake, Dr. Tadashi Ishii, the coordinator for disaster medicine officially appointed by Miyagi's prefecture governor as well as a surgeon from JRC Ishinomaki Hospital, established coordination among various pertinent institutions such as Miyagi's prefecture government, municipal governments of the medical zone, local medical associations, local dental associations, local pharmaceutical associations, Tohoku University Hospital, and JSDF in order to efficiently utilize medical resources with a limited number of medical relief teams.

The Ishinomaki Zone Joint Relief Team was established on March 20, 9 days after the earthquake, so that all medical relief teams could coordinate their relief efforts. It included the Japan Medical Association Team, the Japan Dental Association Team, the Japanese Red Cross relief team, the JSDF Medical Team, the Japan Pharmaceutical Society Team, and other medical relief teams from hospitals all over the country. The joint relief team not only made decisions regarding the day-to-day course of action but also plotted long-term strategies consulting 22 experts of disaster medical care and organizational management from across Japan.

All medical relief teams that came to the Ishinomaki region were registered for participation in the joint relief team (Fig. 10.2).

The medical relief teams began by visiting all emergency shelters to make an initial assessment. The collected information included the number and condition of evacuees, food and water conditions, availability of electricity and water/sewage, access to supplies for warmth such as blankets or heaters, and the sanitary condition of toilet facilities. They finished initial assessments of all shelters in the medical zone ($n = 300$) in 3 days (Fig. 10.1). After receiving the assessments, the Ishinomaki Zone Joint Relief Team task force determined the course of action for each relief team. The relief team collected this information from shelters every time the rounds were made enabling the most effective and updated courses of action to be coordinated with local governments. For example, initial assessments revealed that 35 emergency shelters lacked adequate supplies and that 100 shelters were contaminated by heavy sludge and had unsanitary toilet and water sewage conditions. Miyagi's prefecture government and municipal governments were informed of these conditions so that a solution could be organized.

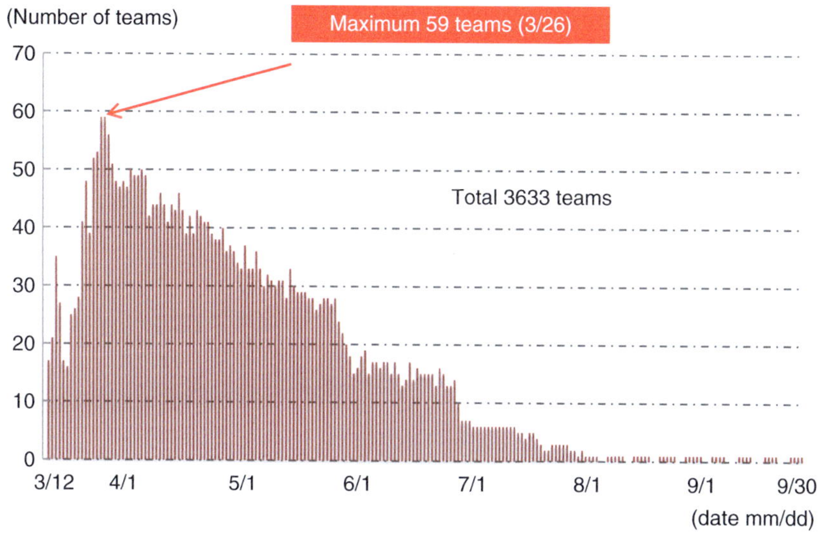

Fig. 10.2 Number of medical relief teams that joined the Ishinomaki Zone Joint Relief Team. On March 26 (15 days after the earthquake), a maximum of 59 teams joined the Ishinomaki Joint Relief Team. Out of the total 3633 teams, 1101 teams were from the JRC Society. The activities of the Ishinomaki Zone Joint Relief Team were completed by the end of September 2011

10.4.3 Welfare Evacuation Centers

The initial surveillance of emergency shelters revealed that 76 refugees who required nursing care had been scattered around different shelters. In order to care for these refugees effectively, they were sent with their families to welfare evacuation centers which had been established at two community halls that had escaped severe tsunami/earthquake damage. Physicians regularly made rounds; nurses, physical and occupational therapists, and nutritionists stayed in these welfare evacuation centers treating and caring for the admitted refugees. Patients requiring nursing care, patients with disabilities, and LTOT patients who had escaped to JRC Ishinomaki Hospital were also transferred to the centers; this made it possible to make rooms available for those patients who could only receive proper treatment at the hospital.

10.4.4 Mobile Dispensing Pharmacy

A temporary dispensing pharmacy was established the day after the earthquake at JRC Ishinomaki Hospital. There, pharmacists and physicians responded to all visiting patients including those who had lost their drug prescription information during the disaster. Unfortunately, many people, especially those who had lived in the more severely affected areas, were unable to reach the hospital. While medical relief teams could bring emergency medication to treat certain symptoms and pains, they could not provide adequate medication that would cover the entire gamut of chronic diseases.

Thirteen days after the earthquake, a movable dispensing pharmacy team, Melon Bread Team, comprised of physicians and pharmacists, was organized. The team went around to the various shelters and inquired patients with chronic diseases about their medical history, current medical condition, and related medication information in order to make the appropriate prescriptions. After pharmacists at JRC Ishinomaki Hospital dispensed the prescriptions, Melon Bread Team or other visiting medical relief teams delivered the prescribed drugs to each shelter.

10.4.5 Infection Control Activity in the Medical Zone

As the center of the Ishinomaki Medical Zone was inundated for several days and the sanitary conditions of many shelters remained very poor (see Sects. 10.4.1 and 10.4.2), the prevalence of infectious diseases such as gastroenteritis, influenza, and other respiratory infections was a serious concern.

Two of the certified infection control nurses from JRC Ishinomaki Hospital were fully engaged in the infection control activity of the medical area. They educated hand hygiene, gargling, health coughing etiquette, etc. to people in shelters, community members, and disaster volunteers. Assessment data of the number of patients with symptoms at shelters and first aid stations by the Ishinomaki Zone Joint Relief Team were updated and monitored daily (Fig. 10.3). The certified nurses were sent to the shelters where there was an increase in the number of patients with symptoms in order to monitor sanitary conditions of the shelters and give advice on infection control.

With the total cooperation of the International Relief Department of the Japanese Red Cross Medical Treatment Center, simple hand-washing facilities were set up at 11 shelters selected based on the assessment. The joint relief task force enlisted the cooperation of contractors to provide 90 wrap-type portable toilets for emergency shelters in the Ishinomaki area that needed them—primarily for the elderly. The Western-style wrap-type toilets (waste is solidified by chemicals for sanitary disposal) not only improved the sanitation of shelters but also put minimal stress on the knees of the elderly.

Fortunately, the medical area did not experience an outbreak of gastroenteritis or influenza during the aftermath of the earthquake (Fig. 10.3).

10.5 External Assistances

During the aftermath of the Tohoku Earthquake, a tremendous amount of human resources and relief supplies were sent to the affected areas by national and international organizations as well as private individuals. In the Ishinomaki Medical Zone, medical relief human resources and supplies were sent mainly to JRC Ishinomaki Hospital.

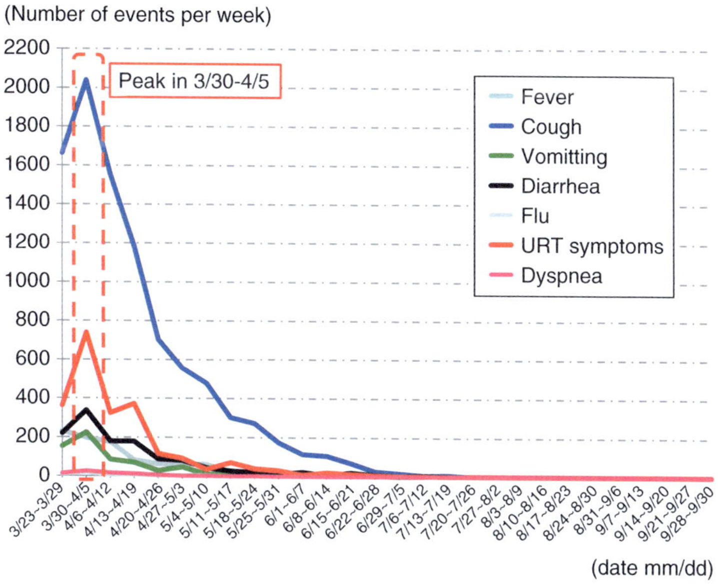

Fig. 10.3 Acute symptoms of refugees at shelters or first aid stations. Cough and upper respiratory tract symptoms had a steep peak from March 30 to April 5. Sunny and windy days during this period aroused thick dust from the tsunami sludge likely contributing to air pollution. This might have further contributed to the significant increase in respiratory symptoms. However, the number of patients exhibiting symptoms of gastroenteritis and influenza did not increase much during the aftermath of the earthquake

Another important source of external assistance came in the form of relocating patients to hospitals or nursing homes outside of the affected areas as described in 10.3.2. This type of assistance significantly reduced the burdens of the healthcare system within the stricken areas.

10.5.1 Medical Relief Team [5]

As described in Sect. 10.4.2, the Japanese Red Cross Society and other nonaffiliated relief teams from all over the country were registered as a part of the Ishinomaki Zone Joint Relief Team. Each relief team stayed and carried out their missions for 4–5 days. By the end of September 2011, 180 days after the Tohoku Earthquake, 3633 relief teams had participated in the joint relief team; 1078 of these relief teams were from the Japanese Red Cross Society, while the remaining two-thirds were from other nonaffiliated relief teams (Fig.10.2).

The coordinating headquarters were set up at the JRC Ishinomaki Hospital. The Ishinomaki Medical Zone was divided into 14 areas based on the distribution of emergency shelters. Several relief teams, each one referred to as a line, were allocated to each area as needed. One of the lines was designated as the managing team in charge of deciding the next day's activity. General meetings were held every evening in order to report the daily activities of the relief teams in each area. The coordinating headquarters assessed emergency medical needs and decided the comprehensive activities of the medical zone.

The medical need for shelters gradually decreased as infrastructure was restored, and local general physicians resumed their clinics. The activities of the joint relief team were completed by the end of September 2011 (Fig. 10.2).

10.5.2 Medical Support of Human Resources for JRC Ishinomaki Hospital

As JRC Ishinomaki Hospital preserved its hospital function after the Tohoku Earthquake, large numbers of victims (the number of emergency patients peaked at 1200 on the third day of the earthquake—60 times more than the hospital's average number of patients) visited the hospital. A minimum twofold increase in the number of emergency patients lasted for 6 months following the earthquake.

The hospital's staff were also affected by the disaster. While nobody on staff was killed, 5% of them lost members of their families, and one third of them experienced significant or complete damage to their houses.

In order to continue disaster medical relief effectively and protect staff from physical and mental health issues, medical support from human resources for the hospital was crucial. The JRC Ishinomaki Hospital received substantial support from a variety of medical specialists including psychiatrists who treated hospital staff members for any potential mental health problems.

The Department of Respiratory Medicine, comprised of five full-time physicians, was nearly overwhelmed by the influx of victims suffering from respiratory diseases. With the help of 1–2 relief respiratory physicians, as well as 3–4 senior and junior residents inside the hospital, the department could continue practicing disaster respiratory medicine without any of the respiratory physicians becoming ill or overfatigued.

However, there were several problems regarding the disaster relief support for the hospital. First, because it took some time to develop the skills necessary for using and interpreting the medical information system and to become accustomed to the work schedule, short-term staff replacements did not work well; 7–14 days of work from staff replacements was desirable. Second, quite a few medical relief members preferred practicing disaster medicine at the front line of the disaster site more than working inside the hospital. Third, extended support from external sources might have led the hospital staff to become heavily dependent on relief support even when the practical need for such support gradually diminished. Thus, relief support for the hospital was withdrawn 5 months after the earthquake.

10.6 Lessons Learned

10.6.1 General

1. A detailed manual that assumes the worst scenario and realistic training conducted on a regular basis were both effective throughout the initial response. During the aftermath of the earthquake, many unexpected complications arose. Most of such difficulties were overcome by applying the risk management cycle [6] and by staff's strong judgment.
2. The integration of information and a unified chain of command were essential in maximizing the efficacy of relief activities during the aftermath of the disaster. For example, it was not quite efficient for each relief team to visit shelters by their own accord or as directed by some organization (see Sect. 10.4.2).
3. Local governments and communities should make efforts to address the ever-changing conditions of relief supply transportation. In places where lots of relief supplies are collected, personnel should keep them organized so that they may be distributed properly and effectively.
4. Disaster base hospitals should also take control of the medical relief supplies throughout their respective areas. They should understand which specific medicines and medical devices are lacking and should transmit the information so that they can receive and distribute proper and timely support.
5. Especially vulnerable populations, such as the elderly or those unable to perform certain activities of daily living (ADL), should be evacuated out of stricken areas as soon as possible. Certain disaster relief agreements regarding the relocation of affected vulnerable people between distant local governments or involving the wide-area hospitality industry might be considered.
6. For an island country like Japan, transportation of relief supplies and relief teams over bodies of water is especially crucial when a large-scale disaster causes widespread destruction of roads. Also, hospital ships are very effective in treating people who have evacuated to coastal area during the aftermath of a catastrophe.

10.6.2 Specific to Disaster Respiratory Medicine

1. The earthquake and tsunami significantly increased cases of respiratory emergencies, especially pneumonia, COPD exacerbation, and asthma attack. Smoking in or near the entrances of the shelters should be prohibited. Dustproof masks should be provided at shelters, communities, and volunteer centers.
2. Refugees receiving LTOT came to JRC Ishinomaki Hospital simply to receive oxygen and stayed there for as long as 15 days (see Sect. 10.3.3). This created a severe strain on hospital bed space and the healthcare staff practicing acute-

phase disaster medicine. Medical care evacuation centers which accommodate patients by providing LTOT should be discussed under peacetime conditions to prepare for a large-scale disaster. An agreement regarding the registration of and assistance for LTOT patients during large-scale disasters was assembled between JRC Ishinomaki Hospital, municipal governments of Ishinomaki Medical Zone, medical associations of the medical zone, and LTOT devices suppliers. The agreement states that (a) LTOT patients will be registered at each municipal government of the medical zone; (b) LTOT centers will be set up at the JRC Ishinomaki Hospital as well as other specified community centers; (c) following the announcement of a large-scale disaster by the JRC Ishinomaki Hospital, LTOT device suppliers will provide the necessary devices to LTOT centers according to instructions by the hospital; and (d) information for LTOT patients about safety and evacuation will be integrated at the hospital.
3. Healthcare professionals should educate patients with chronic respiratory diseases so that they can personally manage their own diseases through practicing the self-management and their individual action plan in ordinary times. Healthcare professionals should also educate patients about general disaster preparedness. In the event of a disaster, people will rarely perform as efficiently and effectively as they do in practice.

10.7 Conclusion

Torahiko Terada, a Japanese physicist and haiku poet, wrote in his essay, "Acquire a sense of fear you need, no less, no more," criticizing mountain climbers who underestimated the dangers of an active volcano. When a human is faced with challenges that he or she has never considered, that person is likely to lose the ability to think and act rationally. Therefore, general preparedness for large-scale disasters and tabletop exercises that simulate the worst possible disaster scenario are essential to surviving a natural disaster.

Acknowledgment The author would like to thank Eunghee Cho for his vigorous proofreading and useful suggestions.

References

1. US Department of Homeland Security National Response Framework. Chapter 2: response action, 42. 2008. http://www.fema.gov/pdf/emergency/nrf/nrf-core.pdf
2. Yamanda S, Hanagama M, Kobayashi S, Satou H, Tokuda S, Niu K, Yanai M. The impact of the 2011 great East Japan earthquake on hospitalization for respiratory disease in advanced aging society: a retrospective descriptive and cross-sectional study at the disaster base hospital in Ishinomaki. BMJ Open. 2013;3:e000865. https://doi.org/10.1136/bmjopen-2012-000865.

3. Kobayashi S, Hanagama M, Yamanda S, Yanai M. Home oxygen therapy during natural disasters: lessons from the great East Japan earthquake. Eur Respir J. 2012;39:1047–8.
4. Japan Defense Focus. Great East Japan earthquake and SDF's activities: special number, 2012. http://www.mod.go.jp/e/jdf/sp2012/sp2012_02.html
5. Ishii T. Medical response to the Great East Japan Earthquake in Ishinomaki City. WPSAR. 2011;2 https://doi.org/10.5365/wpsar.2011.2.4.005.
6. WHO. Rapid Risk Assessment of Acute Public Health Events. http://apps.who.int/iris/bitstream/handle/10665/70810/WHO_HSE_GAR_ARO_2012.1_eng.pdf;jsessionid=862CD4437C815A26716ACB2DD35E873D?sequence=1.

Part IV
Countermeasures Against Disaster for the Patients with Respiratory Diseases

Chapter 11
Anti-disaster Measures in Local Public Entities for Patients Prescribed Long-Term Oxygen Therapy: Have Local Public Entities Made Appropriate Anti-disaster Measures for Patients Prescribed Long-Term Oxygen Therapy?

Keisaku Fujimoto

Abstract It is necessary to develop countermeasures against disasters using the combination of government and private funding drawing on previous experience with large-scale earthquake disasters. Cooperation among multiple disciplines and organizations beyond the affected area is important to develop and improve mutual aid for neighborhoods. However, countermeasures developed to date for patients with respiratory disease, especially those prescribed long term oxygen therapy (LTOT), are no longer sufficient. Not all patients prescribed LTOT are included as subjects requiring assistance during a disaster in most local public entities. This may be due to a low degree of recognition about the reason why patients require oxygen, deficiencies in systems for oxygen supply, and weakness of such systems in the event of a disaster. This chapter discusses the anti-disaster measures implemented over a wide area of Matsumoto City and neighboring cities and villages, which are superior to those in other local public entities in Japan especially with regard to countermeasures for patients prescribed LTOT. In addition, various issues related to the countermeasures for patients prescribed LTOT during a disaster are discussed.

Keywords Anti-disaster measure · Long-term oxygen therapy · Local public entity Matsumoto City · Self-protective organization

K. Fujimoto
Department of Clinical Laboratory Sciences, Shinshu University School of Health Sciences, Matsumoto, Japan
e-mail: keisaku@shinshu-u.ac.jp

K. Fujimoto (ed.), *Disaster and Respiratory Diseases*,
Respiratory Disease Series: Diagnostic Tools and Disease Managements,
https://doi.org/10.1007/978-981-13-2598-4_11

11.1 Lessons of Three Recent Great Earthquake Disasters in Japan

The Great Hanshin-Awaji Earthquake Disaster occurred in March 1995 and resulted in large-scale destruction of buildings and homes, with fires increasing the number of deaths. Japan did not have a dedicated disaster medical care system at the time of this earthquake disaster. This disaster prompted the preparation of disaster center hospitals, disaster medical assistance teams (DMATs), and wide area disaster emergency care information systems. The Great East Japan Earthquake Disaster occurred off the Pacific coast of Tohoku in March 2011, with a death toll of 17,000 people. The tsunami resulting from the earthquake was responsible for the majority of deaths due to drowning and also caused an accident at the Fukushima No. 1 nuclear power plant. This latter aspect of the disaster caused widespread pollution of the surrounding land and sea and disrupted the lives of local residents. The Kumamoto Earthquake disaster occurred in April 2016, directly causing 50 deaths and 175 disaster-related deaths. Large numbers of people were evacuated to temporary refugee accommodations, where many people slept close together on the floor, with some staying in tents outdoors or in their cars because of insufficient anti-disaster measurements. These conditions increased the number of disaster-related deaths, including those caused by acute pulmonary thromboembolism due to deep vein thrombosis (DVT). This chapter discusses the advances in anti-disaster countermeasures in local public entities and introduces the anti-disaster measures implemented over the wide area of Matsumoto City and neighboring cities and villages, which are superior to those in other local public entities in Japan especially with regard to countermeasures for patients prescribed LTOT. The problems with these countermeasures in the Matsumoto area will also be discussed.

11.2 Anti-disaster Measurements in Japan

11.2.1 Disaster Prevention System in Japan

Japanese laws regarding disaster control based on the Basic Act on Disaster Control Measures clarified the authority and responsibilities of government and local public entities in all areas of disaster management, such as prevention, emergency response, recovery, and reconstruction, and disaster measures are taken with a combination of government and private funding [1]. The main point of the Basic Act on Disaster Control Measures consists of the following seven main items: (a) clarification of the concepts and responsibilities for disaster prevention, (b) organization of disaster prevention, (c) disaster prevention plan, (d) promotion of disaster control measures, (e) measures for protection of disaster victims, (f) financial support measures, and (g) emergency response measures for disasters. Item (h) includes the prior collation of lists of people requiring assistance during a disaster and clarification of criteria related to refuge facilities in the event of a disaster. Figure 11.1 shows the construction of the disaster control plan in Japan. The Cabinet Office is responsible for issuing instructions and commands in the event of a major disaster; however, local public entities actually play roles in coordination with business operators.

11.2.2 Cooperation and Responsibilities of Government and Local Public Entities

In the event of a disaster, the city, town, and village governments, which are most familiar to residents, respond to the emergency disaster control measures. The prefecture deals with the disaster when comprehensive processing over a wide area is necessary. The government sets up emergency management headquarters to implement rescue operations, first aid activities, medical activities, and the supply and conveyance of relief supplies and also takes charge of liaison and coordination with the local public disaster entity to gather information about the disaster area, support demands, and implement emergency disaster control measures accurately and quickly based on the needs of victims. It is important for the local public entity to be aware of the presence of people requiring assistance and support during a disaster or an emergency and to understand the specificity of chronic diseases and treatments, such as oxygen therapy and mechanical ventilation at home and dialysis.

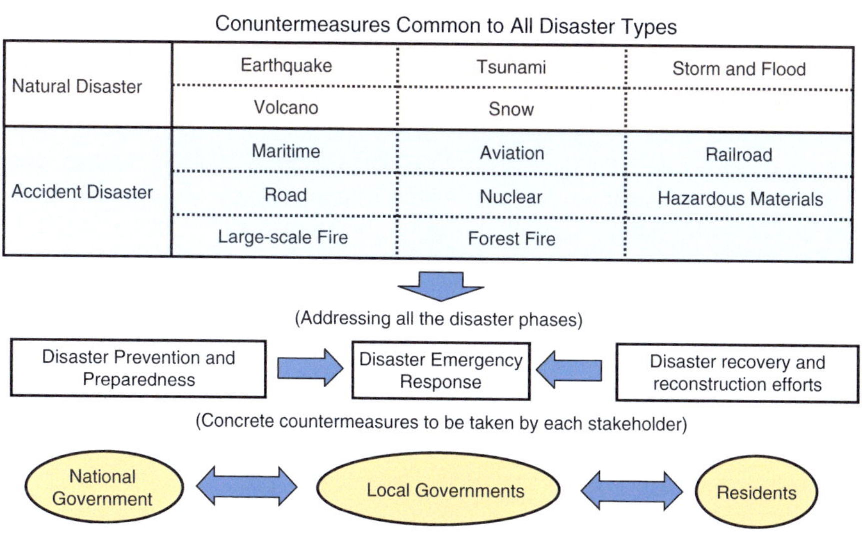

Fig. 11.1 Structure of basic disaster management plan in Japan. From the website of the Cabinet Office: http://www.bousai.go.jp/1info/pdf/saigaipamphlet_je.pdf pp.11, reference [10]

11.3 Have Appropriate Anti-disaster Measures Been Taken for Patients Prescribed Long-Term Oxygen Therapy (LTOT) in Japan?

11.3.1 Results of Questionnaire Survey in 2012 Regarding Correspondence for Patients Prescribed LTOT in a Disaster [2]

From November 2012 through December 2012, Dr. Kida leading the research team conducted a questionnaire survey regarding correspondence for patients prescribed LTOT in the event of a disaster to 1742 local public entities in Japan. A total of 863 local public entities responded (response rate: 50%). A total of 650 local public entities responded "yes" to the question, "In your local public entity, are patients prescribed LTOT classified as people requiring assistance during a disaster?" In 25% of 863 local public entities, patients prescribed LTOT were not specifically classified as people requiring assistance during a disaster. However, among the 650 local public entities that answered "yes," most had restrictions regarding patients prescribed LTOT who were classified for assistance, and only 12% of these local public entities answered that all patients prescribed LTOT were classified as requiring support in a disaster.

Among the restricted conditions, 47% of the 650 local public entities that gave a "yes" response indicated that patients prescribed LTOT were classified for assistance if they had some degree of physical disability and/or had nursing care insurance. Assistance was based on disability in 14% of these local public entities, nursing care insurance in 3%, and other restrictions (such as intractable disease, household with an elderly person, elderly person living alone, etc.) in 24%. Among the criteria for physical disability, 51% of 412 local public entities indicated that assistance was based on a grade > 2. In Japan, the classification of the degree of internal disability does not have grade 2 [3]. The first grade includes patients with severe limitations in activities of daily living due to impairment of pulmonary function, patients who can hardly walk due to severe dyspnea, patients who cannot be evaluated due to severe impairment of pulmonary function, patients with pulmonary dysfunction index (FEV_1/predicted VC) <20%, or those with arterial blood oxygen pressure <50 Torr. According to the white papers regarding respiratory care in Japan in 2005 and 2010 [4, 5], only 36% of patients prescribed oxygen at home, including patients treated with home mechanical ventilation (HMV), had certified > grade 2 disability. That is, only 36% of patients prescribed LTOT in about half of all local public entities were classified as people requiring assistance during a disaster.

The majority (90%) of the 340 local public entities proposed restricting classification of people requiring assistance during a disaster according to the availability of nursing care insurance > grade 3 [6]: i.e., patients requiring assistance with personal care and excretion, patients requiring assistance to transfer to another place and maintain a standing position, and those showing some problematic actions such as loitering and reduced mental capacity. According to the 2010 white paper for respiratory care in Japan [5], among the patients prescribed oxygen at home, including those also prescribed HMV, only 12% had certification of nursing care insurance > grade 3. It may be suggested that the system of LTOT is not understood at all. For the questionnaire item "Please check all organizations that should cooperate in support planning for patients prescribed LTOT in the event of a disaster," the items checked by the largest number of local public entities were the nursing care insurance service (n = 235 of 488 total entities) and physical disability supervision posts of the government office (n = 320 of 488 total entities), followed by welfare service providers (n = 110 of 488 total entities) and fire stations (n = 130 of 488 total entities). Only 33 of 488 local public entities (6.8%) checked oxygen provider as the most important organization for cooperation in support planning for patients prescribed LTOT in the event of a disaster. In addition, 66% of local public entities that responded that patients prescribed LTOT were not classified as requiring special assistance did not have a plan in place for such patients in the event of a future disaster. These results suggested that most local public entities do not recognize or understand the system of oxygen supply.

11.3.2 Questionnaire Survey Among Medical Societies of Wards, Districts, and City

Responses to the survey were received from 657 of 815 wards, districts, and city medical associations in Japan (80.6%). Forty-two medical associations (6.4%) responded "yes" to the question "Has a useful system been built for communication with patients receiving home medical care in an emergency?" Of the 615 medical associations, 5% responded "no" regarding whether they have a concrete plan to build such a system in future; 48.1% responded that they did not have a concrete plan but will consider in future; and 29.8% had no plan and were not taking it into consideration in the future. Among the 42 local medical associations that already had a communication system for use in an emergency, 55.6% replied that they could extract necessary patients from the whole area in the event of an emergency and planned blackouts. It will be necessary to determine the differences among local public entities and medical associations and to understand the weak points of patients prescribed LTOT in the event of a disaster. It will be necessary to immediately develop concrete measures in cooperation with various specialists and areas, such as core hospitals, medical associations, pharmacist association societies, nursing societies, and physical and occupational therapists societies.

11.4 Process of Developing Activities for Rescue and Medical Care Manuals in the Event of a Disaster in Matsumoto City

Matsumoto is located at the center of the Japanese Islands, situated in a basin surrounded by high mountains (the Northern Alps and the Central Alps), with a population of approximately 200,000. The area around Matsumoto includes the Gofukuji Fault, which is part of the Itoigawa-Shizuoka tectonic line fault zone crossing the central part of the Japanese Islands. The probability that a major earthquake will occur within 30 years was increased by approximately twofold from 14% to 25% due to the crustal movement occurring in the East Japan Great Earthquake Disaster. The Earthquake Research Committee estimates that a great earthquake of magnitude (M) 8 will occur in the area in association with the neighboring fault. Preparations for a disaster have been underway for the past 10 years involving cooperation between local public entities and medical societies in Matsumoto City. Matsumoto City in cooperation with Matsumoto-shi medical society has developed a manual of activities for rescue and medical care in the event of a disaster in Matsumoto City itself [7]. In August 2013, the neighboring cities, Azumino-shi and Shiojiri-shi, along with the five villages, Asahimura, Yamagatamura, Ikusakamura, Chikuhokumura, and Omimura, produced a guide for medical cooperation in the event of a disaster (an earthquake with seismic intensity ≥6) in the area surrounding Matsumoto [8].

In 2015, an estimate of the likely damage associated with an earthquake of M 8.5 and maximum seismic intensity 7 along the Itoigawa-Shizuoka tectonic line fault zone in Matsumoto was published. Such a disaster was estimated to result in 1010 deaths, 7940 injured people (4350 with severe injury, 3590 with moderately and mildly injuries), with 88,880 refugees on the second day (36.7% of the population of Matsumoto City) and complete destruction of 24,220 houses. At that time, there was sufficient disaster supplies, such as food, blankets, and corrugated board to make simple temporary beds, for only approximately 5% of the population of Matsumoto City.

11.5 *Manual of Activities for Rescue and Medical Care in the Event of a Disaster in Matsumoto City*, Second Edition [9]

The manual of activities for rescue and medical care in the event of a disaster in Matsumoto City, second edition, emphasized the necessity of cooperation. As the damage will spread beyond the city and villages in the event of a great earthquake, the medical system will require cooperation between the prefecture, city, village, and medical staff (Fig. 11.2). Especially, the city and village governments have a

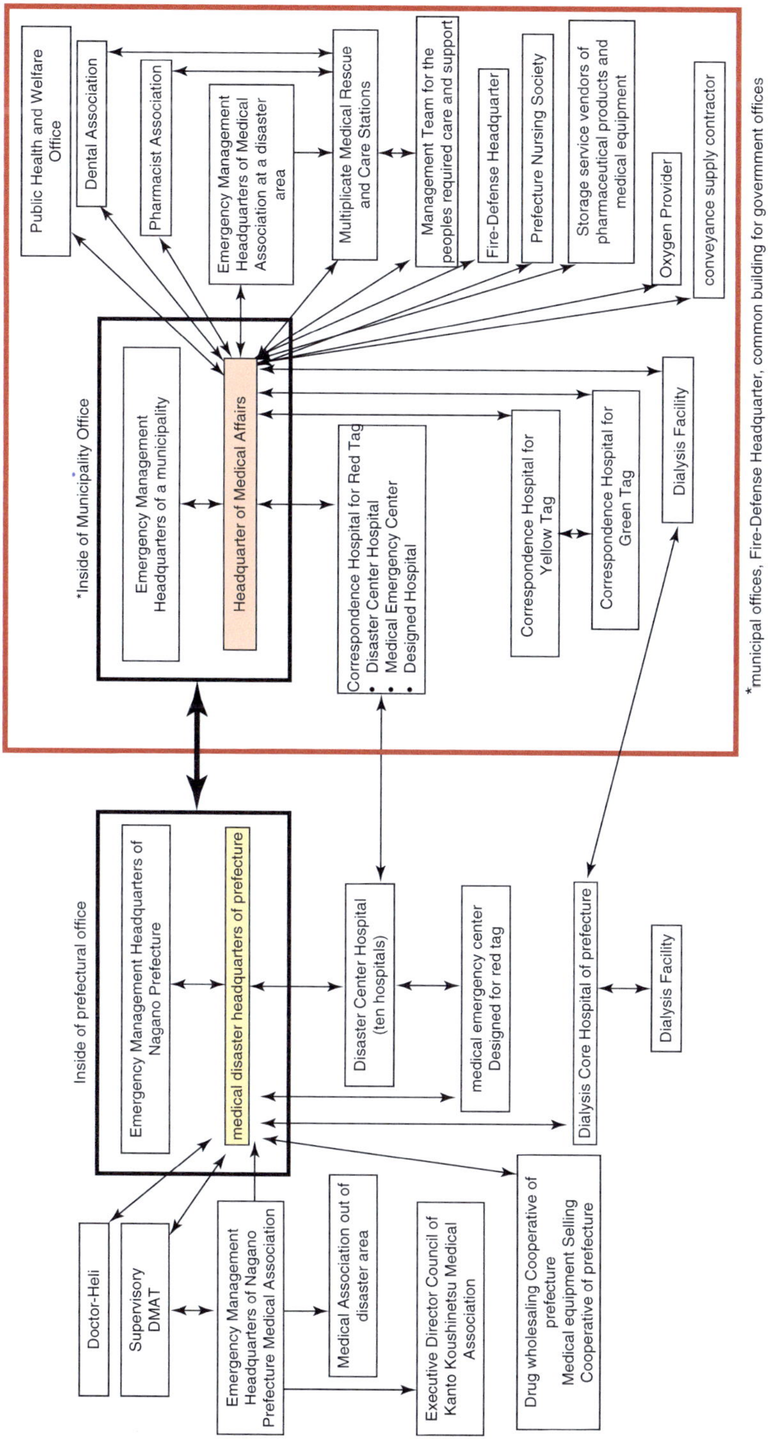

Fig. 11.2 Chart of structure and chain of command in the event of a disaster in Matsumoto City

duty to protect residents' lives, health, and property against a disaster and should carry out anti-disaster correspondence in cooperation with medical staff immediately after the occurrence of a disaster. The following points are important in medical care in the event of a disaster: (a) establishment of the chain of command, (b) maintenance of information transmission network and communication network tools, (c) establishment of refuges and first aid stations, (d) triage of the sick and wounded according to severity, (e) transportation of the sick and wounded within the area, (f) acceptance to a designated disaster center hospital, (g) maintenance of a conveyance base to the outside area (Shinshu Matsumoto Airport) and transportation, (h) measurement for people requiring assistance during a disaster, and (i) development of power of residents for self-management and assistance of vulnerable persons within the neighborhood.

In addition to top priority cases, such as peoples with severe physical/intellectual disabilities and in-home elderly people requiring grade 3–5 nursing care, the support plan highlighted the following as those in need of safety confirmation in the event of a disaster: patients with intractable diseases, parents to care for young children, pregnant women, foreign nationals, people with dementia, the elderly living alone, patients prescribed LTOT, and dialysis patients. All of these people should be registered, either by themselves or by their family, in the registration system. Despite appeals to residents by the local public entities, not all of the people requiring assistance during a disaster register due to concerns over personal information security. A survey performed in 2016 suggested that there are approximately 44,000 (18.3%) people that would require assistance during a disaster in Matsumoto City, including 451 patients prescribed LTOT. In the area of Matsumoto City and neighboring cities and villages, the number of people requiring support is estimated to be approximately 82,903, including 947 patients prescribed LTOT [10] (Table 11.1).

11.6 Medical Support for People Requiring Assistance During a Disaster

The following four points have been proposed for support under normal conditions (i.e., not during a disaster): (a) maintenance of a registered list of people requiring assistance in the event of a disaster (including patients prescribed LTOT and hemodialysis patients), (b) awareness of the need for giving priority to support of people requiring assistance, (c) developing a support system for daily life and establishing rescue and medical care systems (self-protective organization), and (d) reinforcement of the activity of the support team by the refuge governing board on the basic principle of the self-protective organization. The self-protective

Table 11.1 Estimated number of the peoples requiring assistance during a disaster in a wide area of Matsumoto city and neighboring two cities and five villages

One's house (conveyance) ⇒ screening at the prior refuge (conveyance) ⇒ receiving facilities		
Kind of person requiring assistance during a disaster	Number of persons	Responsible Department
Physical disability	4379	Disability Welfare Division
Mentally handicapped	634	
Severe psychosomatic disabled person	115	
Mentally handicapped person	975	
Patients with intractable diseases	1847	
Pregnant and parturient women	1908	Health Support Division
Parent for cradling their baby	8108	
In-home aged persons needing nursing care of grade 3–5	4155	Aged Welfare Division
Dementia	9610	
Elderly peoples who live alone	7809	
Foreigner	3710	Division of Human Rights Sexual Symbiosis
Patients prescribed LTOT	451	Hospital responsible patients treated with LTOT
Dialysis patient	608	Aizawa Hospital
Total amount	44,309	

Data in 2016 of 242,000 population of Matsumoto City [10]

organization is an organization formed by residents based on mutual aid in protecting life, health, and property of residents and to minimize damage occurring in the event of a disaster. The self-protective organization is comprised of town organization units, of which Matsumoto City has a total of 493, some of which are combined into 35 district town cooperative societies (Fig. 11.3). The chairpersons of these 35 district town cooperative societies comprise the Matsumoto City Alliance Society. Thus, the organization has three levels of structure. In addition, each town unit has a number of organizations, such as an assembly, group, and neighborhood association. The town unit is an area community, which is the most familiar to residents and carries out activities associated with the life of residents. Each town unit has posts, including town chairperson, vice-town chairperson, accounts, and various specialized sections, such as hygiene, welfare, and disaster prevention. The town organization runs a public hall. A refuge is prepared by each town unit for use in the event of a disaster, and the public hall is usually designated as a refuge that gives priority to people requiring assistance during a disaster as distinguished from general refugees. In addition, a self-protective organization reports confirmation of the safety of residents to the support team immediately after the occurrence of a disaster.

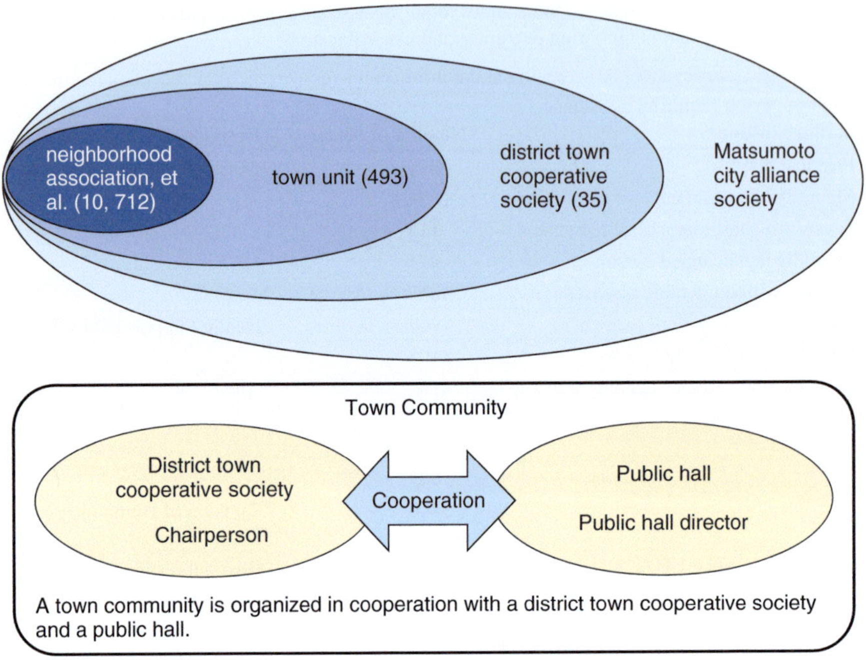

Fig. 11.3 Three-layer town assembly structure in Matsumoto City

11.7 Reinforcement of Support for Patients Prescribed LTOT

The requirements for calculation of medical treatment fees for LTOT include the following: (a) securing of a hospital to which patients can be admitted in an emergency, (b) explanation of emergency oxygen therapy, and (c) explanation of management in an emergency, including at night, with means of communication with an oxygen provider in an emergency. However, 41.5% of the patients prescribed LTOT replied "yes" to the question "Have you ever received an explanation of management in an emergency, such as a disaster?" However, 35% of the patients replied "no" to this question. The remaining 23.5% replied uncertain. More than of the half patients who answered "yes" had received an explanation from an oxygen provider. It is necessary to ensure that the attending physician is aware of the necessity of explaining correspondence and preparations for emergencies and disasters to patients prescribed LTOT.

In addition, the manual indicates that both the attending physician and oxygen provider should carry out the following items in the event of a disaster:

(a) Provide advice to patients prescribed LTOT to register as people required assistance in the event of a disaster.

(b) Provide guidance regarding the breathing method in an emergency to effectively utilize limited oxygen and to ensure the availability of spare oxygen cylinders.
(c) Oxygen providers should make and distribute a card common throughout the Matsumoto wide area indicating patients prescribed LTOT in cooperation with each medical association and should ensure that the patients know how to take action in the event of a disaster. In addition, local public entities of the three cities and five villages in the Matsumoto area should deal with the adjustment of oxygen providers.
(d) Attending physicians (of each medical association) should adjust the appointed hospital for admission in the event of a disaster (however, this will be difficult for the attending physicians because they should go to the medical rescue station in charge).
(e) Oxygen providers establish a system for cooperation with each local public entity of cities and villages under normal conditions, confirm their safety, check the situation of oxygen generator operation, and immediately bring LTOT equipment to homes, appointed places of refuge, or home oxygen therapy centers (HOTC) in the event of a disaster. However, it will take more time to confirm patient safety.
(f) Each medical association and oxygen provider should start and run an HOTC in coordination with a medical team at the headquarters in each of the three cities. The conditions to select a location for the HOTC are as follows: (1) availability of an emergency power supply generator, (2) when it is possible to isolate infectious diseases from general refugees, and (3) ability to prepare sufficient water, food, and heating equipment in winter.
(g) Plan to start an HOTC at two sites in Matsumoto City, one site in Shiojiri City, and one site in Azumino City (elementary and high schools do not fulfill conditions a, b, and c), with management by neighborhood medical facilities. In the five villages, patients prescribed LTOT will be taken to the associated hospital by helicopter or car.
(h) Among the patients prescribed LTOT, the patients prescribed at the flow rate between 3 and 5 L/min and those prescribed at a flow rate of $\geq$ 5 L/min should be admitted to each appointed hospital accompanied by their family, e.g., by car, while those prescribed at a flow rate of $<$ 3 L/min should go to the HOTC.

11.8 Importance of Preparation for a Disaster Under Normal Conditions

It may be necessary to make preparations to ensure that patients will have a power supply until municipal power can be restarted (assuming 3–5 days). A battery is insufficient, and although expensive it is important to ensure availability of a power supply generator.

11.8.1 For Patients Treated with HMV

It is important to secure availability of sufficient batteries in consultation with a medical equipment manufacturer and to ensure that patients are familiar with the use of an artificial nose instead of a humidifier and manual ventilation using a bag valve mask under normal conditions in preparation for the time of an emergency. In addition, the patients or their family should build associations to ask neighbors for help.

11.8.2 For Patients Prescribed LTOT

The following points are important for patients prescribed LTOT. (a) Confirmation of the oxygen requirements or the required minimum oxygen flow rate in an emergency by asking to the attending physician. (b) Confirming with the attending physician whether intermittent inhalation and temporary reduced quantity of oxygen are possible. (c) Confirming whether the oxygen concentrator has a battery function. (d) Securing a portable oxygen cylinder and an oxygen cylinder for emergency use. (e) Preparing actions to take in the event of an emergency, such as calmly changing to an oxygen cylinder if an oxygen concentrator is not available. (f) Manifesting the contact information to oxygen provider at emergency clearly. (g) Considering use of a portable oxygen concentrator that can be charged from a car.

Anti-disaster drills, including measures for patients prescribed LTOT, have been performed at least once a year in Matsumoto City (Fig. 11.4).

11.9 Problems of the Anti-disaster Measures in Matsumoto City

(a) Not all of the people requiring assistance in the event of a disaster are included in the registration system due to concerns regarding personal information protection, and further appeals for active registration by the attending physicians and medical staff are necessary. In addition, the attending physician and medical staff are not always informed regarding the situation of registration, and this is dependent on the report from the patient.
(b) It is doubtful whether all of the people requiring assistance during a disaster, their families, and other residents have been provided with sufficient information about the *Manual of Activities for Rescue and Medical Care in the Event of a Disaster in Matsumoto City* Second Edition and wide area of Matsumoto City and neighboring cities and villages and how many patients prescribed LTOT recognize or have received an explanation about anti-disaster measures. It is important to provide the information to all residents.

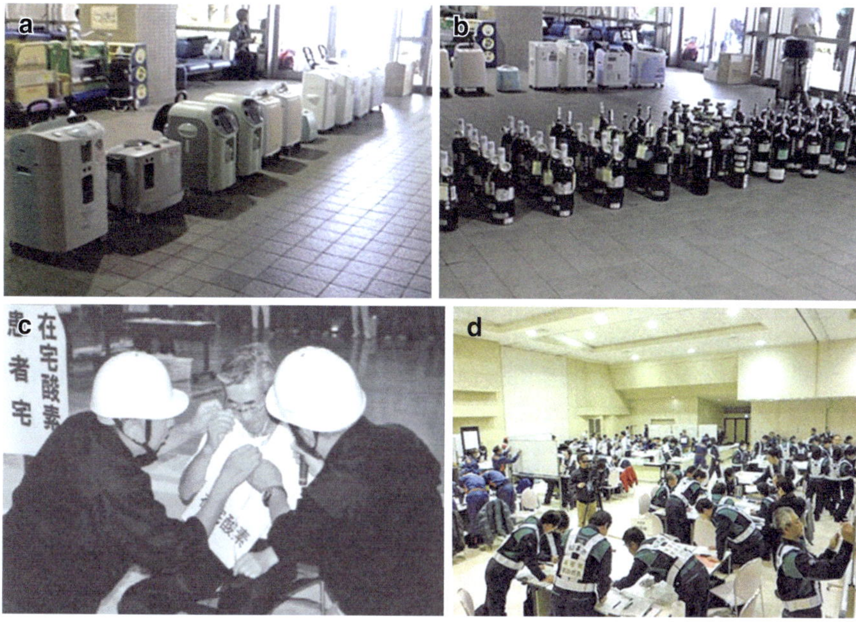

Fig. 11.4 Anti-disaster drill in Matsumoto City. Oxygen concentrators (**a**) and portable oxgen cylinders (**b**) were gathered in the home oxygen therapy center (HOTC). (**c** and **d**) show the drill

(c) It is difficult to determine the appropriate site to open the HOTC. It is difficult to secure power supply in an emergency, to isolate from general refugees, and to prepare beds at the refuge. Therefore, it may be better to set up the HOTC at a medical center, such as a hospital, but this suggestion has not yet been accepted.

(d) Patient information among oxygen providers has not yet proceeded sufficiently, and information sharing and the cooperation system have not yet been fully implemented.

(e) Problems remain regarding the lack of development of the residential environment for refugees in the subacute and chronic periods immediately after a disaster not only for patients prescribed LTOT. For example, corrugated cardboard beds and cooperation systems with healthcare facilities for the elderly have not been fully prepared due to funding shortages.

(f) There is concern about the performance of self-protective organization in the event of a disaster. The personal information of people requiring assistance during a disaster is usually given to the chairpersons of the district town cooperative society and the neighborhood association, but it is not clear whether they understand the situation regarding the necessity of assistance and support and the specificity of treatment with LTOT. There are large differences in the attainment of anti-disaster measurement in the event of a disaster in each district town society. Actually, the concrete action in the event of a disaster is not yet planned completely in most of district town society and neighborhood. Currently, the

correspondence to the patients prescribed LTOT is dependent on the oxygen providers grasping the situation of the patients.
(g) There is concern regarding the replacement of members, aging, and decrease in number of houses in the district town society, as well as how many people will be able to play a role in an emergency situation and that voluntary disaster prevention may malfunction due to a lack of qualified people.

11.10 Conclusion

Anti-disaster measures are dependent on each local public entity, and there are marked differences in measures implemented among each local public entity. Particularly, measures for patients prescribed LTOT are insufficient. In addition, concrete measures for patients who develop pulmonary infectious diseases or acute thromboembolism due to deep vein thrombosis (DVT) and aggravation of chronic lung diseases, such as asthma and COPD, induced by deterioration of the residential environment (i.e., refuge environment) or stopping the supply of medicine and medical equipment have not been made. The anti-disaster measures in Matsumoto City including the neighboring cities and villages may be improved by proactively producing manuals and guidelines for behaviors in the event of a disaster, and all of the patients prescribed LTOT should be classified as people required assistance during a disaster. However, many problems remain. It is obvious that not only medical staff can respond to a disaster, and cooperation with multiple disciplines and multiple organizations is required, such as other local public entities outside the area, core hospitals, medical institutions, fire stations, medical associations, pharmacist societies, nursing societies, dental associations, suppliers of pharmaceutical products and medical equipment, oxygen providers, home care service stations, transportation companies, and self-protective organization. In addition, it is important to promote the development of support systems in cooperation with government to improve the neighborhood mutual aid capacity. This may improve the capacity for self-help where supporters interact proactively with people requiring support. It is important to develop a support system that corresponds to the area.

References

1. Disaster Management in Japan. 3-2 Disaster management plans 2. The Disaster Management System. http://www.bousai.go.jp/1info/pdf/saigaipamphlet_je.pdf. pp.11.
2. Fujimoto K, Sakai S. Questionnaire survey in 2012 about the preparation of support system for the peoples required assistance during a disaster in local public entities of Japan concerning with the response to the patients prescribed long-term oxygen therapy at an emergency and disaster. Reports from the research group of Ministry of Health and Welfare. 2013. pp. 18–26.
3. Health and welfare services for the persons with disabilities. In: Home page of ministry of health, Labor and Welfare. http://www.mhlw.go.jp/english/policy/care-welfare/welfare-disabilities/index.html

4. Japanese White Paper on Home Respiratory Care: Summary. The Japanese White Paper on Home Respiratory Care Production Committee (Fukuchi Y, Kawashiro T, Mishima M, Fujimoto K, Ishihara H, Miyamoto K, Tatsumi K, Ueki J). Edited by Japanese Respiratory Society, Tokyo. 2006.
5. Japanese White Paper on Home Respiratory Care 2010. The Japanese Respiratory Society and the respiratory failure research group from the Ministry of Health, Labor, and Welfare, Japan, Medical Tribune Co. Ltd, Tokyo. 2010.
6. Long-term care system in Japan. In: Home page of Ministry of Health, Labor and Welfare. http://kensaku.mhlw.go.jp/search?q=system+of+long-term+care+insurance&btnG=search&site=mhlw_collection&client=mhlw_frontend_E&proxystylesheet=mhlw_frontend_E&output=xml:no_dtd&ie=utf-8&oe=utf-8
7. Manual of activities for rescue and medical care at the time of a disaster in Matsumoto city, 2nd edn. Matsumoto City Official Website: https://www.city.matsumoto.nagano.jp/kurasi/bosai/torikumi/bosai_keikaku/iryou/iryoukyuugo_manual.html
8. Guidance of Medical Cooperation at the time of a disaster in a wide area zone of Matsumoto city and neighborhood cities and villages- it will be applied when an earthquake with a seismic intensity of a lower 6 or greater occurs.). Publication: Disaster Medical Care Conference in Wide Area of Matsumoto, Matsumoto, August 2013.
9. Fujimoto K. Problems concerning with the response to the patients prescribed long-term oxygen therapy at an emergency and disaster in Matsumoto City. Reports from the research group of Ministry of Health and Welfare. 2014. pp. 22–26
10. Medical care system at a disaster in the future- for all at the time. In Suzawa H. (Ed.). Matsumoto City: Medical Association, Matsumoto. 2016.

Chapter 12
Anti-disaster Measures for Patients: What Measures Can Patients Take to Prepare for Disasters?

Takashi Motegi

Abstract The elderly are generally vulnerable and prone to suffering in the aftermath of a disaster. Moreover, older patients with chronic respiratory diseases likely experience continuous symptoms such as dyspnea or asthma attacks. Among such patients, those receiving therapy for long-term oxygen or home ventilation become the first victims of a calamity. Family members, medical staffs, and employers belong to local governments are equally requested additional task or rescue compared with those people during the disaster. However, patients have to take their own steps in order to make a decision, with or without assistance. It was reported that patients who had attended educational training offered by hospitals before the Great East Japan Earthquake disaster were better able to manage their daily activities than those who had not. This chapter describes anti-disaster measures that patients can take to prepare for calamities through joint daily practice with family members and hospital staff, based on experiences from recent earthquakes that have struck Japan.

Keywords Self-management · COPD · Self-help · Action plan

12.1 Introduction

Japan has a long history of natural disasters, including frequent earthquakes, volcanic eruptions, floods, and typhoons. The 2011 Great East Japan Earthquake (GEJE) was the greatest natural disaster to hit Japan after the Second World War and led to the greatest loss of life and number of people missing: approximately 20,000 casualties. Those over the age of 60 accounted for 66.1% of deaths [1]. The vulnerability of the elderly during this crisis was a serious problem [2] in terms of policy.

T. Motegi
Respiratory Care Clinic, Nippon Medical School, Tokyo, Japan
e-mail: mo-dr@nms.ac.jp

K. Fujimoto (ed.), *Disaster and Respiratory Diseases*,
Respiratory Disease Series: Diagnostic Tools and Disease Managements,
https://doi.org/10.1007/978-981-13-2598-4_12

During the initial stages of a disaster, all people need to protect themselves (i.e., engage in self-help). Seventy-two hours following a calamity, local communities can offer mutual help. Central and local governments might also have a chance to provide aid to the public victims equally. In general, public help is not likely to be available immediately after a disaster (such as within 24 h), although partial relief efforts might begin at that time. According to a government survey [3], during the Great Hanshin Earthquake of 1995, neighborhood families and residents rescued 70% of survivors, including rescuing people trapped under debris from collapsed buildings. However, groups such as firefighters, police, and the Japan Self-Defense Forces only rescued 30% of the victims.

In general, the oldest senior citizens (those over 85 years old) are more likely to have deteriorated health conditions with various chronic diseases (including cognitive disorders) and might have a fair amount of difficulty helping themselves during a disaster. Nevertheless, all people—including those who are very vulnerable—should develop the ability to take care of their own needs. From the experience gained from the GEJE, it can be stated that medical staff should incorporate training of patients in self-management into their daily practice, thus maximizing patients' ability to utilize self-help. Thus, all possible victims can be trained to handle any type of disaster.

In order to implement preventive actions into daily routines, patients with chronic obstructive pulmonary disease (COPD) probably comprise the best sample for this purpose. The impacts of COPD on individuals' health and ailments are related to the quality of life and entail huge medical expenses; COPD is currently the third leading cause of death worldwide. Even in patients with mild to moderate COPD, most of them experience frequent cough, sputum and dyspnea on exertion, or asthma attacks, even under stable conditions. Currently, some clinical phenotypes of COPD have shown frequent exacerbation, rapid deterioration and/or a decline in the activities of daily living (ADL) with reduced lung function, and many comorbidities. Recent clinical guidelines of COPD [4] indicate that daily management and prevention of exacerbation are fundamental for disease control. Current research has focused on suitable interventions for self-management education [5]. Education on the self-management of daily living is vital, especially during a disaster's initial or prolonged phases.

In this chapter, based on a patient survey conducted after GEJE, we describe how patients with COPD learned to practice countermeasures that would help them take care of their essential needs in the event of a disaster.

12.2 Comprehensive Flow of Disaster Countermeasures Based on Time

Comprehensive disaster countermeasures usually consist of four phases: (1) mitigation, (2) preparedness, (3) response, and (4) recovery [6]. Mitigation is used to minimize subsequent social disorder. Preparedness involves planning concrete countermeasures at the individual, group, and regional levels, and teaching individuals how to take necessary actions in case of a disaster. These two phases are conducted during normal times and their contents overlap, but both are undertaken before a calamity strikes. Response countermeasures are initiated immediately after a disaster. Recovery countermeasures describe the process followed to return to normal conditions after the chronic phase of a disaster ends. The response and recovery stages begin after a disaster. In other words, the four phases have two counterparts: before and after.

These four phases are applied to patients with COPD. During the mitigation phase, the impairment factor of patients who have problems before and after a calamity is identified, and educational training specific to their disease is offered to them as well as to their families. As part of preparedness, disaster measures are developed for each patient. At this time, it is also useful to create an action plan that can be implemented when a calamity has not yet occurred. This plan includes evacuation drills, such as verifying the locations of evacuation centers and actually going there. Response measures include protecting oneself first, evacuating immediately after a calamity, continuing necessary medical care, taking steps to prevent the spread of infectious diseases, and ensuring that one has access to adequate food and water. The recovery process involves returning to normal life for an extended period and engaging in physical activities, monitoring disease progression, and avoiding complications (see Fig. 12.1).

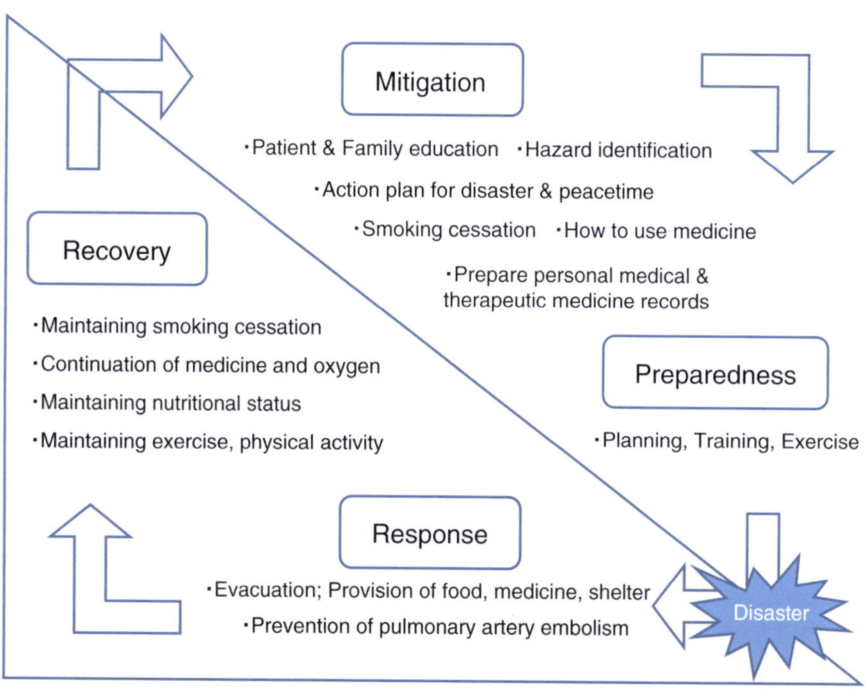

Fig. 12.1 Disaster phase and patients with chronic respiratory disease

Table 12.1 Medical and patient movement from disaster occurrence to termination

	Phase 0	Phase 1	Phase 2	Phase 3	Phase 4
	Just after 6 h	6–72 h	72 h–1 week	1 week–1 month	1–3 months
Medical phase	Immediately after the disaster	Hyper-acute stage	Acute stage	Sub-acute stage	Chronic stage
Medical activity	*Activities of DMAT *Relief from outside the region *Establishment of medical counterpart *Establishment of evacuation center, medical aid, and medical aid stations				
Patient's conditions and behavior	*Protect oneself; secure personal safety *Confirm safety; contact stakeholders *Wait in a safe house; move to an evacuation center *Make contact with medical personnel; prevent complications				

DMAT disaster medical assistance team

The process that begins immediately after a disaster and ends when conditions have returned to normal is divided into further phases. At each stage, time axes represent the movement of patients and medical staff (see Table 12.1). The axes summarized in this table are based on the data from the Tokyo Metropolitan Disaster Medical Council and Tokyo Metropolitan Welfare and Health Bureau [7].

Phase 0 lasts until 6 h after the disaster. Rescues and related activities are initiated when many sick people have been affected, and fires, collapsed buildings, or other kinds of impacts have injured individuals. A disaster medical assistance team (DMAT) is formed immediately after the disaster, and activities commence. During this phase, it is necessary for patients to take steps to protect themselves, and for others to assess and act in a way that helps the largest number of people and families. Safety confirmation will be done after personal safety has been secured.

The hyper-acute phase occurs between 6 and 72 h afterward. During this phase, the number of patients being transported to medical institutions increases, but there are also disruptions to lifelines and transportation, and there is little human or physical support from sources outside the afflicted area. Medical triage assessments of patients' conditions begin. At this stage, patients are moved to a safe place or evacuation center. Ambient aids are also often required.

The acute phase lasts from 72 h to 1 week after the disaster. Damage is assessed, lifelines are restored, and a system for receiving support is established. Patients begin to be transferred to facilities outside the disaster zone, where more appropriate medical interventions are available.

The sub-acute period lasts from 1 week to 1 month after the disaster. Lifelines, transportation, and other facilities are gradually restored during this time. Beginning at this stage, cases of pneumonia, COPD, and asthma are exacerbated, and preventive medical interventions become necessary. Patients need to practice good hygiene to prevent infection, should continue to engage in physical activity, and should be aware of the increased risk of contracting a secondary illness.

The chronic phase lasts from 1 to 3 months and marks the stage during which the lives of those who have been evacuated are stabilized. The focus shifts to coping with chronic ailments rather than providing acute care. During this time, healthcare workers engaged in disaster areas are medical personnel who can cope with chronic diseases.

In the medium to long term—3 months after the disaster—many aspects of daily life have returned to normal. The usual medical system has nearly been resumed. Mental care and support associated with the disaster are also continued.

Based on the history of disasters, it is mainly during the initial stage that patients, their families, and local residents (self-help/co-assistance) take direct action in response to the crisis. Once people have been evacuated and their safety ensured, medical personnel (co-assistance/public assistance) determine where they will be placed. For medical staff, the question is what pre-education patients themselves require beforehand that will help them during future calamities.

12.3 Preparing for a Disaster: Self-Management Education

In terms of chronic respiratory diseases, the self-management education approach to COPD has been the one most studied. The aim of self-management through medical intervention is ultimately to achieve health effects by changing patients' behavior. As part of this process, it is necessary to increase patients' self-efficacy through medical interventions and create a situation in which it is easy to alter one's behavior.

During self-management interventions, patients and medical personnel need to interact. "These patient-centered interactions focus on: (1) identifying needs, health beliefs and enhancing intrinsic motivations; (2) eliciting personalized goals; (3) formulating appropriate strategies (e.g., exacerbation management) to achieve these goals; and if required (4) evaluating and re-adjusting strategies" [5]. Patients' needs are stressed because people are more effective when they are motivated to learn and feel the necessity of doing so.

The perspective of practicing self-care during disasters is basically similar to normal times, but it is not easy to promote the need for disaster countermeasures during normal times. It is difficult for patients and doctors to actively work on such steps if they do not feel the need to do so. How can a patient with a chronic illness be expected to do what is difficult even for a healthy person?

It may be more effective to provide opportunities for guidance by simulating disaster scenarios, such as those patients themselves are likely to face in the future. While patients and medical staff are sharing actual disaster information, they can discuss the actions that will be necessary in the future. Both patients and medical staff need to acknowledge that what we cannot do normally will not be possible in the event of a disaster.

12.4 Respiratory Patients' Problems During the Great East Japan Earthquake

The Japanese Red Cross Ishinomaki Hospital (JRCIH) took on the central roles of the Ishinomaki medical area during GEJE. According to the JRCIH report, many patients had pneumonia or experienced an exacerbation of COPD within several days of the disaster. The decline in the ADL of elderly people became prominent

Table 12.2 Problems that occurred in patients with respiratory diseases due to the Great East Japan Earthquake

Acute phase	Lost or lacked medicine
	Oxygen became unusable
	Could not move to the shelter
	Lack of food and water
	The evacuation destination was unknown and could not be contacted
	Could not explain one's illness
	Could not explain one's prescribed medicine
	Could not explain one's oxygen flow rate
	Symptoms worsened due to discontinuing drugs and oxygen
	Exacerbation
	Nutritional status could not be maintained
	Could not keep exercising
	Could not go home since one's house had collapsed
Chronic phase	Daily living activity declined

when their evacuation exceeded 3 weeks [8, 9]. Although the incidence of respiratory diseases increased immediately after GEJE, which is not surprising, the report noted that the way in which survivors are affected after evacuating must also be considered. Table 12.2 lists the problems patients faced after the earthquake.

The JRCIH had been developing an educational system for patients with COPD prior to GEJE, and these effects were examined after the disaster [10]. According to the JRCIH report, about 106 people with COPD (50 affected by the disaster, 56 not affected) were able to continue their exercise therapy after the earthquake (70% of the affected patients and 87% of the patients not affected by the disaster). The percentage of patients who suffered from dust inhalation included 70% of those impacted by the disaster and 98% of those not affected. It was speculated that survivors who were not able to continue with their exercises lost access to medical treatment due to the crisis. Subsequent JRCIH surveys revealed that patients' self-care education greatly contributed to their self-management after the disaster [10]. This exemplifies a situation in which mutual assistance was provided in a well-structured hospital that is supportive of patients. However, this response was possible only because the staff were very well trained. These problems are discussed, and the points of self-management are detailed in the next section.

12.5 Disaster Countermeasures for Patients on Home Oxygen Therapy

12.5.1 Japan's Medical System

Japan's medical system is different from those in Western countries such as the USA, and it is necessary to know these differences before the discussion. All Japanese citizens receive the same medical insurance through the central government, and in many cases, patients pay only 10–30% of the total cost of treatment, including diagnostic tests and medications. A restriction on the number of visits is warranted to guarantee that medical institutions can provide services to all citizens. One more characteristic of Japan's medical system is free access that allows patients to see any doctor they wish in a medical facility. If a patient's need for home oxygen therapy falls under the qualification criteria, treatment is covered by public insurance. Although an oxygen provider delivers the oxygen device to the patient's home, the patient does not pay the provider directly for the medical costs associated with the device. Insurance qualifications require that patients who need oxygen therapy receive monthly visits and management by their doctors at each medical institution. Since oxygen therapy is provided in this way, oxygen companies play a relatively significant role in the medical system, even during disasters, in addition to the roles played by patients and medical staff [11].

12.5.2 How Patients on Oxygen Therapy Cope During Disasters

12.5.2.1 Who Needs Assistance?

According to a survey administered to the patients registered with Japan's patients' association of respiratory diseases (650 people, with an average age 73.2 years, 65.7% of whom are male), 360 of these individuals (55.4%) had previously experienced at least one disaster, and most of them had gone through the earthquake [10]. When asked whether there was a need for assistance in the event of a calamity, 322 people (49.5%) said there is always a need, 140 people said it depends on the time and occasion, and 125 people (19.2%) said they did not need help. Patients who said they needed some kind of assistance were older, were severe cases, had more shortness of breath, and required home oxygen therapy or used a ventilator.

12.5.2.2 Preparing Patients to Use Disaster Countermeasures

Only 215 patients (33.1%) had cards that provided instructions on what they should do in an emergency. In terms of confirming the locations of evacuation sites during a disaster, 336 (54.6%) patients knew how to arrive at their evacuation sites and had actually gone there, while only 94 (15.3%) had verified the route. Eighty-one patients (13.2%) had not confirmed where their evacuation sites were and said they would not know what to do during a future disaster. For this reason, many patients responded by saying, "I cannot evacuate due to shortness of breath" or "I cannot go to an evacuation center with an oxygen cylinder."

In the survey of patients requiring home oxygen therapy, 45.3 and 54.0%, respectively, were not able to explain how they would cope with difficulty breathing or with a panic attack. One hundred sixty-nine (39.5%) could not explain how to use the medical equipment provided to them for long-term oxygen therapy, or the ventilators, which could not be used during a power outage [10].

12.5.2.3 Problems with the Patient Support System

In Japan, primary care physicians treat many patients requiring home oxygen therapy. The cost of oxygen therapy is covered by medical insurance, but it is hard to say he/she is receiving good-quality medical care, and preparedness planning for domestic patients is very limited. Medical institutions should offer instruction and education for patients requiring oxygen therapy. In practice, however, there is a possibility that providing this education would depend on oxygen suppliers. We should clearly document what content medical staff should teach patients. The failure to provide prior guidance to patients becomes a serious problem once a disaster occurs.

12.6 What Is Necessary Self-Management Education Before and After a Disaster?

The contents of the self-management education required for chronic respiratory diseases, including COPD, are roughly divided into six categories [12]: (1) understanding the disease, (2) medication therapy, (3) exercise therapy, (4) nutritional therapy, (5) guidance to quit smoking, and (6) exacerbation management. For each category, the required content is summarized for both normal times and disaster/recovery periods (see Fig. 12.2).

These are the basic requirements to assist patients with respiratory diseases, but there are also measures specific to disasters that should be taught to all patients, regardless of their illness. These include self-management behaviors immediately after the disaster and evacuation drills beforehand.

Quitting smoking: Quitting smoking is the most basic treatment for respiratory diseases. However, patients who stop smoking may start again due to the stress caused by a disaster. It is necessary that the provided support will enable patients to refrain from smoking after a disaster. Psychological interventions such as stress management are also necessary.

Understanding disease: It is desirable for patients to understand the physiology and pathology of their diseases to some extent. They should be aware of the possibility that their condition may deteriorate in the event of a disaster and try to prevent this as much as possible. In the case of poor physical health, medical personnel should be contacted promptly. At the time, the goal will be to have the patient explain their illness to some extent. Patients should also prepare a disaster prevention notebook and record information about their ailments.

Drug therapy: The patient should understand the purpose of the medication prescribed and how to use it. In the event of an emergency, there is a possibility that the

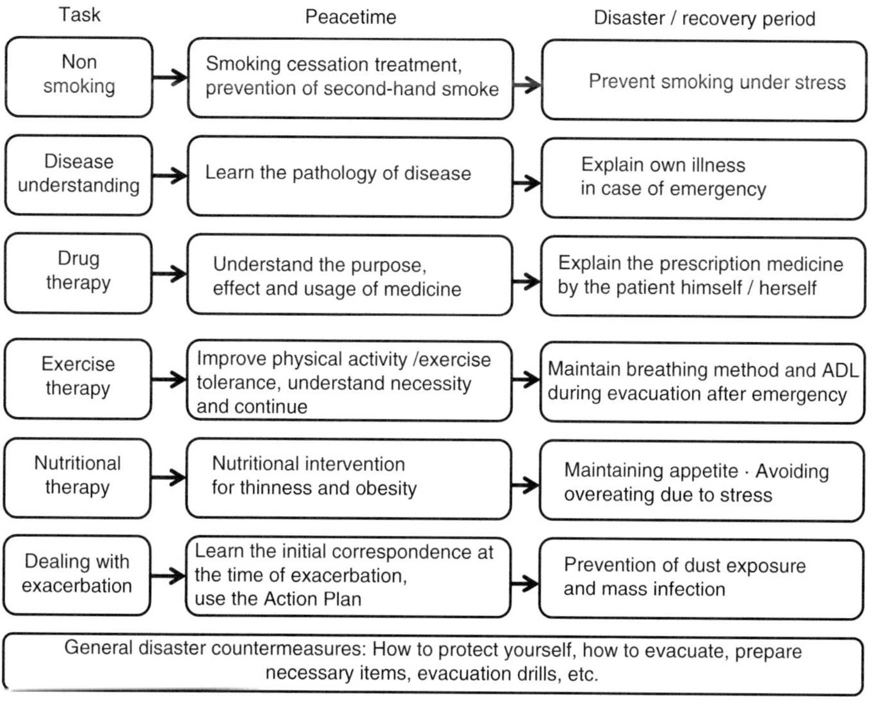

Fig. 12.2 Self-management contents during peacetime, disaster, and recovery in respiratory disease patients

medical treatment received until then will be suspended or canceled. For patients with chronic diseases, medical staff should be informed that treatment should be continued, even in the event of a disaster [13]. By having patients record their own prescriptions in a medication notebook, original prescriptions could be continued based on this record, even after a calamity strikes [14].

Exercise therapy: Patients should be taught why exercise rehabilitation is necessary when there are no disasters. Specific instructions should be given on the content and frequency of exercise. Patients should also be taught to practice pursed-lip breathing, even after an emergency and evacuation, so as to enable them to move their bodies as much as possible. During GEJE, one patient who experienced respiratory rehabilitation taught pursed-lipped breathing to other patients who had no prior experience using it. This is a good example of how patients can provide mutual assistance to their peers. When living as evacuees, the risk of lower limb vein thrombosis develops due to insufficient bodily movement. To prevent this condition, we instruct patients to make time to be moderately active, even when living at an evacuation site.

Nutrition therapy: Patients should be educated on why obesity and leanness are problems, and they should have a dietician teach them about specific diets. Encourage them to stockpile several days' worth of food and drinking water in advance of an unexpected crisis. Also note the dietary environment after the disaster and pay attention to food poisoning that might be caused by an unsanitary environment.

Coping with and preventing disease exacerbation: Patients should be taught to use the action plan for their initial correspondence in the event that their illness worsens. After exacerbation has been dealt with, preventive measures they can take in the future should be discussed. Patients should be encouraged to wear masks to avoid inhaling the dust that increases after a calamity and practice thorough hand-washing, since viral infections tend to spread when people live in shelters. Influenza or pneumococcal vaccines should be used to inoculate patients if they qualify according to the situation.

Countermeasures specific to disasters that are common to all diseases: There is a possibility that patients themselves may be forced to practice self-help for 3 days after a disaster. There is usually a lack of immediate outside help; therefore, patients need to consult with their medical doctors beforehand about what they should do. Ideally, they would prepare an action plan that would clarify how they should act (Fig. 12.3).

Items that will be needed during a disaster, including medicines, should be prepared and kept ready. It would be best to have a reserve of prescriptions that will last several days to a week. According to a report on the delivery system of a wholesaler of medicines to medical institutions/pharmacies in the disaster area after GEJE, except for the center of the disaster, 70% or more of delivery functions were restored by the third day after the earthquake, and over 90% of delivery functions were recovered within 1 week [15].

Patients should confirm the locations of the designated evacuation centers in their residential areas. As much as possible, they need to know to arrive at their

Disaster Action Plan

- Act calmly
- Take a position to protect yourself
- Make sure that you are safe now
- Move to a safe place
- Prepare the necessary medicines
- Carry a personal medicine notebook
- Contacts (family / friends / emergency number__________)
- Carry valuables, insurance cards, mobile phones
- Carry a spare battery

(For oxygen user)

- Switch to a portable cylinder when a power failure occurs
- Your oxygen flow rate is set to ( ) L/min
- Write the evacuation destination in the memo and leave it in the entrance

Fig. 12.3 Example of a disaster action plan

evacuation sites and verify the routes to take there under normal conditions. Evacuation drills have great value in that it is possible to understand in advance what is likely to pose a problem when a patient moves to an evacuation site.

Family guidance helps patients who usually have difficulty with self-management. Patients living alone are instructed to register with the support services available in their residential area. They should make arrangements to ensure that the assistance they would need during a disaster, such as help moving to a shelter, has been prearranged.

12.7 Disaster Countermeasures for Seriously Ill and Oxygen Therapy Patients

12.7.1 Daily Preparations

List essential requirements: Make a list of the items required in an emergency and stockpile them. Include food and water for at least 3 days, emergency toilets, and pharmaceuticals.

Confirm arrangements/contact methods for aid: After a disaster, seriously ill people will require help moving and relocating to the evacuation site, so arrangements must be made clarifying who will help them and how. When deeming that assistance will be necessary at the time of a disaster, tell patients how they should go about requesting public support from local governments. Beforehand, provide the oxygen vendor with information about the patient's evacuation destination, as well as contact information.

Learn how to use oxygen equipment: In addition to patients, caregivers should be taught how to exchange cylinders. Not all oxygen cylinders at a patient's home should be used up, and there should always be a spare cylinder. Tell patients how long an oxygen cylinder can be used by teaching them about usage flow rates. Make preparations for standby power supply and spare portable cylinders for seriously ill patients requiring an oxygen flow rate of 3 L/min or more during normal times.

12.7.2 Practice Disaster Prevention Drills

Since problems are clarified by allowing patients to act, it is advisable to practice the following training before a disaster:

Change the oxygen: Have patients check how much time is available on the cylinder. Even in the dark, let the patient practice by exchanging the oxygen cylinders and equipment.

Go to the shelter: Confirm the travel route to the shelter and the time required to get there. Let patients go to the evacuation centers with their families. Have the patients put on their backpacks and walk to the site while holding the cylinder. Ask them to review whether there were any problems.

12.7.3 What Patients Needing Oxygen Should Do in the Event of a Disaster

Take action to protect themselves: Patients should move to a safe position immediately after a disaster. If patients need immediate help, they should use a whistle or light to attract the attention of others in the area.

Switch oxygen equipment: Switch to the oxygen cylinder if there is a power outage and oxygen equipment becomes unusable. Check the amount of oxygen remaining in the cylinder and how many remaining cylinders are at hand. If there is no cylinder and no oxygen available, rest as much as possible, and wait to be rescued while consuming less oxygen.

Evacuation and contact: If the patient has plenty of time, have him/her get in touch with a predetermined contact. When moving to a shelter, post information on the individual's evacuation destination at the entrance, so that people who make inquiries later on will know where to find them. Depending on the situation, it may be possible to secure the individual's safety while waiting at home.

Early detection of exacerbation: Since health conditions can worsen quickly due to environmental changes, consult with a staff member or medical professional if an individual's symptoms become altered.

12.8 Disaster and Education Systems from the Angle of the Social System

Since the number of elderly people in Japan will rise in the future, it is necessary to reform the social system in anticipation of a rapid increase in the demand for medical and nursing care. Therefore, the government's goal is to implement a new, comprehensive regional care system (the Integrated Community Care System) by 2025 that will provide autonomous unified medical care, nursing care, and living support services within each region. In essence, this system can be described as building a system to keep living in a familiar town.

With regard to disaster prevention, not only are individuals and families significant but connections with neighboring residents are also important. Reports from previous crises have provided examples of local residents' successful and often lifesaving efforts. It is appropriate to initiate disaster prevention measures within the regional comprehensive care system because the active associations of local communities provide support and assistance during normal times, as well as during calamities [16].

Although difficult to realize, the ideal following a disaster is to build a community that is healthier than the previous one [17]. Disaster response preparations are required for housing, medical facilities, roads, and parks; these kinds of places are not sufficiently integrated into the system. Cohesive measures are needed to jointly prepare residents, medical facilities, and municipalities. From the perspective of patient education, treatment policies need to be unified among medical personnel, and the support system must allow nonspecialists to manage oxygen to some extent. Cooperation with local oxygen companies is needed in addition to oxygen therapy and medical institutions. In the event of a disaster, sufficient oxygen equipment must be secured.

12.9 Conclusion

All patients should practice the following as disaster countermeasures. First, during normal times, they should learn about their ailment from medical staff with knowledge of their illness and obtain advice on treatment measures. They should think about how they could continue to receive the same treatment after a disaster, participate in disaster prevention drills as much as possible, and try to move their bodies. If a patient cannot do this alone, the patient's family needs to participate and prepare for an emergency situation. Since it is difficult to initiate new, unfamiliar activities suddenly after a disaster has occurred, it is essential that we prepare for this eventuality gradually every day.

References

1. Cabinet Office. Government of Japan. Annual report on the aging society. 2013. http://www.cao.go.jp/. Accessed 31 Mar 2018. (In Japanese).
2. Aldrich N, Benson WF. Disaster preparedness and the chronic disease needs of vulnerable older adults. Prev Chronic Dis 2008;5(1). http://www.cdc.gov/pcd//issues/2008/jan/07_0135.htm. Accessed 31 Mar 2018.
3. Cabinet Office Japan, White paper disaster management in Japan 2017. http://www.bousai.go.jp/kyoiku/panf/pdf/WP2017_DM_Full_Version.pdf. Accessed 31 Mar 2018.
4. Global strategy for the diagnosis, management, and prevention of chronic obstructive pulmonary disease. 2018 report. http://goldcopd.org/wp-content/uploads/2017/11/GOLD-2018-v6.0-FINAL-revised-20-Nov_WMS.pdf. Accessed 31 Mar 2018.
5. Effing TW, Vercoulen JH, Bourbeau J, et al. Definition of a COPD self-management intervention: international expert group consensus. Eur Respir J. 2016;48:46–54.
6. U.S. Department of Veterans Affairs. Disaster life cycle: four phases of comprehensive emergency management. Washington, DC. 2002.
7. Bureau of Social Welfare and Public Health. Tokyo Metropolitan Government http://www.fukushihoken.metro.tokyo.jp/iryo/kyuukyuu/saigai/saigaiiryoukyougikai.files/zenbun.pdf. Accessed 31 Mar 2018. (In Japanese).
8. Kobayashi S, Hanagama M, Yamanda S, et al. The impact of a large-scale natural disaster on patients with chronic obstructive pulmonary disease: the aftermath of the 2011 Great East Japan Earthquake. Respir Invest. 2013;51:17–23.

9. Yamanda S, Hanagama M, Kobayashi S, et al. The impact of the 2011 Great East Japan Earthquake on hospitalisation for respiratory disease in a rapidly aging society: a retrospective descriptive and cross-sectional study at the disaster base hospital in Ishinomaki. BMJ Open. 2013;3:e000865.
10. Kida K, Motegi T. Disaster countermeasure of patients with chronic respiratory disease: Information for team approach. Medical Review Co., 2016. Osaka, Japan (In Japanese).
11. Kida K, Motegi T, Ishii T, et al. Long-term oxygen therapy in Japan: history, present status, and current problems. Pneumonol Alergol Pol. 2013;81:468–78.
12. Hyland ME, Jones RCM, Hanney KE. Information needs in COPD patients: the lung information needs questionnaire. Airways J. 2005;3:142–4.
13. Arrieta MI, Foreman RD, Crook ED, et al. Insuring continuity of care for chronic disease patients after a disaster: key preparedness elements. Am J Med Sci. 2008;336(2):128–33.
14. Okumura J, Nishita Y, Kimura K. Pharmaceutical supply for disaster victims who need chronic disease management in region with aging population based on lessons learned from the Noto Peninsula Earthquake in 2007. Yakugaku Zasshi. 2008;128:1275–83.
15. Japanese Pharmaceutical Association. Activity report on the Great East Japan Earthquake. Japanese Pharmaceutical Association, Tokyo. 2012. http://www.nichiyaku.or.jp/press/wp-content/uploads/2012/03/120308_3.pdf. Accessed 31 Mar 2018. (In Japanese).
16. Ministry of Health, Labour and Welfare. http://www.mhlw.go.jp/file/06-Seisakujouhou-12300000-Roukenkyoku/0000165560.pdf.
17. Tuckson RV, Dzau VJ, Lurie N. Creating healthy communities after disasters. New Engl J Med. 2017;377:1806–8.

MIX
Papier aus verantwortungsvollen Quellen
Paper from responsible sources
FSC® C105338

If you have any concerns about our products,
you can contact us on
ProductSafety@springernature.com

In case Publisher is established outside the EU,
the EU authorized representative is:
Springer Nature Customer Service Center GmbH
Europaplatz 3, 69115 Heidelberg, Germany

Printed by Libri Plureos GmbH
in Hamburg, Germany